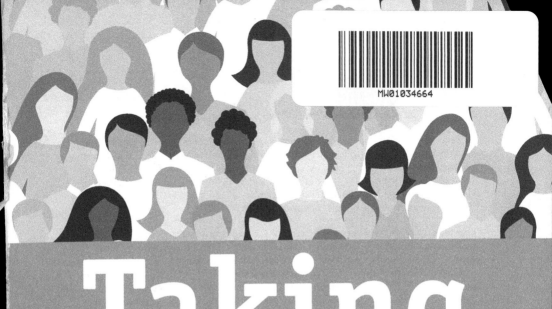

Taking Action

Top 10 Priorities to Promote Health Equity and Well-Being in Nursing

Susan B. Hassmiller, PhD, RN, FAAN
Gaea A. Daniel, PhD, RN

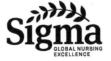

Sigma
GLOBAL NURSING
EXCELLENCE

Sigma Theta Tau International Honor Society of Nursing (Sigma) is a nonprofit organization whose mission is developing nurse leaders anywhere to improve healthcare everywhere. Founded in 1922, Sigma has more than 135,000 active members in over 100 countries and territories. Members include practicing nurses, instructors, researchers, policymakers, entrepreneurs, and others. Sigma's more than 540 chapters are located at more than 700 institutions of higher education throughout Armenia, Australia, Botswana, Brazil, Canada, Colombia, Croatia, England, Eswatini, Ghana, Hong Kong, Ireland, Israel, Italy, Jamaica, Japan, Jordan, Kenya, Lebanon, Malawi, Mexico, the Netherlands, Nigeria, Pakistan, Philippines, Portugal, Puerto Rico, Scotland, Singapore, South Africa, South Korea, Sweden, Taiwan, Tanzania, Thailand, the United States, and Wales. Learn more at www.sigmanursing.org.

Sigma Theta Tau International
550 West North Street
Indianapolis, IN, USA 46202

To request a review copy for course adoption, order additional books, buy in bulk, or purchase for corporate use, contact Sigma Marketplace at 888.654.4968 (US/Canada toll-free), +1.317.687.2256 (International), or solutions@sigmamarketplace.org.

To request author information, or for speaker or other media requests, contact Sigma Marketing at 888.634.7575 (US/Canada toll-free) or +1.317.634.8171 (International).

ISBN: 9781646482023
EPUB ISBN: 9781646482030
PDF ISBN: 9781646482047
MOBI ISBN: 9781646482054

Library of Congress Control Number: 2022951554

First Printing, 2023

Publisher: Dustin Sullivan
Acquisitions Editor: Emily Hatch
Development Editor: Jill Leeper Sycamore
Cover Designer: Rebecca Batchelor
Interior Design/Page Layout: Rebecca Batchelor
Indexer: Larry D. Sweazy

Managing Editor: Carla Hall
Publications Specialist: Todd Lothery
Project Editor: Carla Hall
Copy Editor: Todd Lothery
Proofreader: Erin Geile

Dedications

To my mother, Jacqueline Wouwenberg, one of the first expert nurse clinicians to battle through the polio epidemic and my first and most important role model as a nurse. And to all the nurses around the world who have risen to the occasion to put patients first during the COVID-19 pandemic. So many sick, so many deaths, even among our ranks, yet you do not give up. Strong voices have arisen among you, and new leaders have been forged. Never forget the difference you are making in the lives you are touching.

–Sue Hassmiller

To my mother, whose unconditional love and support continue to call me to dream big. I am who I am because of you. To my husband, whose encouragement and sense of humor always help me get through challenging times. Thank you for your love and patience. To my ancestors, who were never afforded the opportunity to showcase their brilliance to the world. Your sacrifices created the path for my journey.

To the nurses who have been the voices of those who were silenced; who have sacrificed time with family to care for others; who have advocated for equitable, comprehensive healthcare; and who have dedicated their life's work to the pursuit of optimal health for all whom they encounter. I honor you.

–Gaea Daniel

About the Authors

Susan B. Hassmiller, PhD, RN, FAAN, is Senior Advisor for Nursing Emerita at the Robert Wood Johnson Foundation (RWJF). She is the founder and Principal of Sulu Coaching and Consulting (www.sulucoaching.com), with a practice focused on healthcare leaders, and a Hudson/ICF-certified Executive/Leadership Coach. Hassmiller is a national leader in nursing, health equity, and leadership development. She has devoted her career to strengthening the nursing profession, improving population health, and advancing health equity. During her 25 years at RWJF, she served as the Senior Advisor for Nursing and the Senior Scholar-in-Residence/Senior Advisor to the President at the National Academy of Medicine (NAM). She helped to lead the landmark reports at NAM on the future of nursing—*The Future of Nursing: Leading Change, Advancing Health* (2010) and *The Future of Nursing, 2020–2030: Charting a Path to Achieve Health Equity* (2021). She also established and served as the Director of The Future of Nursing: Campaign for Action, a nationwide initiative led by AARP, the AARP Foundation, and RWJF, to transform health and healthcare through nursing to build a healthier America.

Hassmiller has held leadership positions in some of the nation's most prominent healthcare organizations. She served on the Board of Governors of the American Red Cross, is an elected member of NAM, and is a Fellow in the American Academy of Nursing, where she holds Living Legend status. She sits on other advisory committees and boards, including Hackensack Meridian Health System, UnitedHealth Group, Carrier Clinic, the Nurses on Boards Coalition, and the University of North Carolina School of Nursing. She has received many awards and four honorary doctorates, including the Florence Nightingale Medal, the highest international honor given to a nurse by the International Committee of the Red Cross. She lives in Cary, North Carolina, with her husband and close to her extraordinary grandchildren.

Gaea A. Daniel, PhD, RN, is Assistant Professor at the Nell Hodgson Woodruff School of Nursing at Emory University. Daniel is a nurse scientist whose program of research focuses on understanding the sociocultural and environmental influences that affect sexual health behaviors and outcomes. She is particularly interested in sexual health outcomes of Black women that present as race-based disparities, from intravaginal practices to sexually transmitted infections. Daniel is a two-time Robert Wood Johnson Foundation Scholar, selected for both the New Careers in Nursing and Future of Nursing Scholars programs. She is also a Gilead Sciences Research Scholar and an Emory Building Interdisciplinary Research Careers in Women's Health (BIRCWH) Scholar.

Daniel devotes her time to diversity-related initiatives in research and the nursing profession as the Diversity Committee co-chair of the Georgia Nursing Leadership Coalition and the co-founder of the High School to Higher Education Program, which seeks to increase the representation of Black men in nursing. She also enjoys volunteering in the community with the Atlanta Black Nurses, where she serves as the National Institutes of Health's All of Us Research Program Champion. Additionally, she works with SisterLove, Inc., to promote sexual health and positivity in minoritized and underserved communities.

Daniel received her PhD in nursing from Emory University, a master of science in nursing from Augusta University, and a bachelor's degree from Mercer University. She lives in Atlanta, Georgia, with her husband, and enjoys traveling and spending time with loved ones.

Contributing Authors & Artists

Kupiri Ackerman-Barger, PhD, RN, CNE, ANEF, FAAN, is Associate Dean of Health Equity, Diversity and Inclusion and Clinical Professor at the University of California Davis Betty Irene Moore School of Nursing, and Director of Faculty Development for Education and Co-Director for the Interprofessional Teaching Scholars Program for UC Davis Health. *The Who, What, How, and When of Nursing Workforce Diversity*, Chapter 2, p. 25.

Ravenne Aponte, BA, BSN, RN, is currently a doctoral student at the University of Pennsylvania School of Nursing in the Barbara Bates Center for the Study of the History of Nursing and co-creator of Nurses You Should Know. *Nurses You Should Know: Inclusive Storytelling Designed to Expand the Nursing Narrative*, Chapter 10, p. 197.

Gaurdia Banister, PhD, RN, NEA-BC, FAAN, is Executive Director of the Institute for Patient Care at Massachusetts General Hospital and Director of the Yvonne L. Munn Center for Nursing Research. *Now, More Than Ever, Diversity Matters*, Chapter 3, p. 61.

Cynthia Barginere, DNP, RN, FACHE, is Chief Operating Officer of the Institute for Healthcare Improvement. *A Personal Journey to Improving Maternal Health*, Chapter 4, p. 72.

Cyrus Batheja, EdD, MBA, BSN, RN, PHN, FAAN, is National Vice President of Strategic Initiatives, Health Equity and Enterprise Transformation for UnitedHealthcare. *Health-Related Social Needs: Acknowledging and Impacting National Inequities*, Chapter 4, p. 69.

David C. Benton, PhD, RN, FFNF, FRCN, FAAN, is Chief Executive Officer of the National Council of State Boards of Nursing. *Demographics, Diversity, Education, and Health Outcomes*, Chapter 2, p. 29.

Kathryn C. Booth, DNP, RN, CNL, is currently Manager of Emergency Medical Services and Disaster Preparedness at Advocate Illinois Masonic Medical Center. *Disaster Response: Helping Those Who Help Others*, Chapter 6, p. 115.

J. Margo Brooks Carthon, PhD, APRN, FAAN, is Associate Professor of Nursing and Africana Studies at the University of Pennsylvania and co-founder and Executive Director of THRIVE in the Penn Health System. Afterword, p. 205.

Shawna Butler, MBA, RN, is creator and host of the *See You Now* podcast, Managing Director of the Exponential Medicine Conference, and Director of Experience for the Digital Orthopaedics Conference San Francisco. *Technology as a Health Equity Lever*, Chapter 7, p. 129.

Billy A. Caceres, PhD, RN, FAHA, FAAN, is Assistant Professor of Nursing at the Columbia University School of Nursing. *Harnessing the Power of Nursing to Improve Care Delivery for Vulnerable Populations*, Chapter 4, p. 79.

Lucinda Canty, PhD, CNM, FACNM, is a certified nurse-midwife and Associate Professor in the Elaine Marieb College of Nursing at the University of Massachusetts Amherst, provider at Planned Parenthood of Southern New England, host of web discussion *Overdue Reckoning on Racism in Nursing,* and founder of Lucinda's House, a Black maternal health collective. Poetry and artwork, pp. 21, 42, 65, 83, 105, and 126.

Silvia H. De Bortoli Cassiani, PhD, MSC, RN, is Regional Advisor for Nursing and Health Technicians at the Pan American Health Organization/World Health Organization. *Region of the Americas: Health Systems and Nursing,* Chapter 9, p. 175.

Garrett K. Chan, PhD, RN, APRN, FAEN, FPCN, FNAP, FCNS, FAANP, FAAN, President and CEO of HealthImpact, a California nursing workforce and policy center, and Associate Adjunct Professor at the University of California, San Francisco. *Taking Advantage of a Crisis to Forge New Multi-Sector Collaborations,* Chapter 5, p. 98.

Pamela F. Cipriano, PhD, RN, FAAN, is President of the International Council of Nurses and Professor at the University of Virginia's School of Nursing and Batten School of Leadership and Public Policy. *Nurses Caring for Their Communities Around the World,* Chapter 9, p. 170.

Robin Cogan, MEd, RN, NCSN, FAAN, is a nationally certified school nurse in the Camden City School District, the New Jersey State School Nurses Association Director to the National Association of School Nurses, a Johnson & Johnson School Health Leadership Fellow, and faculty in the School Nurse Certificate Program at Rutgers University-Camden School of Nursing. *Pandemic School Nursing—Another Front Line,* Chapter 10, p. 195.

Yvonne Commodore-Mensah, PhD, MHS, RN, FAAN, FAHA, FPCNA, is Associate Professor at the Johns Hopkins Schools of Nursing, Johns Hopkins Center for Health Equity, and Department of Epidemiology at the Johns Hopkins Bloomberg School of Public Health, and a Fellow and board member of the Preventive Cardiovascular Nurses Association. *Nurses as Champions for Global Health Equity,* Chapter 9, p. 167.

Martha A. Dawson, DNP, RN, FACHE, FAAN, is Associate Professor at the University of Alabama at Birmingham School of Nursing, President of the National Black Nurses' Association, and serves on the advisory board for Direct Relief Health Equity Fund. *Resiliency, a Double-Edged Sword: Improving the Culture and Climate of Nursing,* Chapter 8, p. 155.

Vernell P. DeWitty, PhD, MBA, RN, is Chief Diversity and Inclusion Officer at the American Association of Colleges of Nursing. *One Strategy to Increase Nursing Workforce Diversity,* Chapter 3, p. 53.

Bruna Moreno Dias, MSC, RN, is a consultant for the Pan American Health Organization in the Health Systems and Services Department and a PhD candidate at the University of São Paulo – Brazil. *Region of the Americas: Health Systems and Nursing,* Chapter 9, p. 175.

Casimiro Canha Cavaco Dias, MPH, MBA, is the Pan American Health Organization Advisor, Health Systems and Services, for Jamaica, Bermuda, and the Cayman Islands. *Region of the Americas: Health Systems and Nursing*, Chapter 9, p. 175.

Regina Eddie, PhD, MSN, RN, is Assistant Professor in the School of Nursing at Northern Arizona University and an enrolled tribal member of the Diné (Navajo) Nation of Arizona. *A Tool to Promote Cultural Humility to Advance Academic Success for American Indian/Alaska Native Nursing Students*, Chapter 2, p. 38.

Whitney Fear, MSN, PMHNP-BC, is a nurse practitioner at Family HealthCare, a board member for the Indigenous Association, Chairwoman of the Fargo Native American Commission, and an enrolled member of the Oglala Sioux Tribe. *Building Social Capital in Nursing: Doing With Intention*, Chapter 1, p. 5.

Mary Joy Garcia-Dia, DNP, RN, FAAN, is Program Director, Nursing Informatics, Information Technology Department at New York-Presbyterian and adjunct faculty at the Frances Payne Bolton School of Nursing at Case Western Reserve University and the City University of New York School of Professional Studies. *Technology Improvements to Promote Digital Health Equity*, Chapter 7, p. 139.

Treyce Gladney, MBA, is Director of Social Determinants of Health & Health Equity at UnitedHealthcare. *Health-Related Social Needs: Acknowledging and Impacting National Inequities*, Chapter 4, p. 69.

Rosa Gonzalez-Guarda, PhD, MPH, RN, CPH, FAAN, is Associate Professor at Duke University School of Nursing, Co-Director of the Community Engagement Core for Duke's Clinical Translational Science Institute, and an executive member of LATIN-19 (Latinx Interdisciplinary Network for COVID-19). *Mentoring Minoritized Nursing Students in an Anti-Racist Era*, Chapter 3, p. 58.

Wallena "Lena" Gould, EdD, CRNA, FAANA, FAAN, is CEO of the Diversity in Nurse Anesthesia Mentorship Program, Vice Chair of the American Academy of Nursing Diversity & Inclusivity Committee, Co-Chair of the American Association of Nurse Anesthetists Education and Innovation Committee, and Visiting Assistant Professor at the University of South Florida College of Nursing. *Students Who Look Like Me*, Chapter 3, p. 45.

Ernest Grant, PhD, DSc(h), RN, FAAN, is President of the American Nurses Association and adjunct faculty for the UNC-Chapel Hill School of Nursing. *This Is a Journey: Dismantling Structural Racism*, Chapter 1, p. 3.

Lauran Hardin, MSN, RN-BC, CNL, FNAP, is a Senior Advisor for the Illumination Foundation and nurse representative and Vice Chair of the US Government Accountability Office's Physician-Focused Payment Model Technical Advisory Committee. *Addressing Health Equity Together*, Chapter 5, p. 101.

Zenobia Harris, DNP, MPH, RNP, is Co-Chair of the Little Rock Branch of the American Association of University Women and Executive Director of the Arkansas Birthing Project, a mentoring and empowerment program for pregnant

African American women. *Preparing for Disasters and Public Health Emergencies,* Chapter 6, p. 119.

Patricia Ingram-Martin, MS, RN, is Chief Nursing Officer in the Ministry of Health and Wellness of Jamaica and Chair of the RNB Education Sub-committee. *Region of the Americas: Health Systems and Nursing,* Chapter 9, p. 175.

Favorite Iradukunda, PhD, RN, is Assistant Professor at the Elaine Marieb College of Nursing, University of Massachusetts Amherst. *Redistribute Power Over Data, Definitions, and Decision-Making,* Chapter 1, p. 12.

Julius Johnson, DNP, RN, FNP-BC, FAANP, is Associate Professor, Chair of Faculty Affairs, and Director of the Family Nurse Practitioner Program at Long Island University – Brooklyn's School of Nursing and serves as the President of the Greater New York City Black Nurses Association. *Improving Healthcare by Meeting People Where They Are,* Chapter 4, p. 76.

Paule V. Joseph, PhD, MS, FNP-BC, CRNP, FAAN, has a dual appointment as Chief of the Section on Sensory Science and Metabolism in the Division of Intramural Clinical and Biological Research at the National Institute on Alcohol Abuse and Alcoholism and at the National Institute of Nursing Research, and Director of the African Research Academy for Women. *Unmute Us: The Power of Diverse Voices in Nursing & Leadership,* Chapter 10, p. 187.

Taynin Kopanos, DNP, FNP-BC, FAANP, is Vice President of State Government Affairs for the American Association of Nurse Practitioners, where she oversees the state advocacy program. *Going Together,* Chapter 5, p. 89.

Marion Leary, MPH, MSN, RN, is Director of Innovation at the University of Pennsylvania's School of Nursing, a member of the American Nurses Association's Innovation Advisory Committee, a founding member of the Society of Nurse Scientists, Innovators, Entrepreneurs and Leaders, and host of the University of Pennsylvania School of Nursing podcast *Amplify Nursing. Innovation Approaches to Increasing Equity and Decreasing Harm,* Chapter 7, p. 143.

Melina Lopez, BSN, RN, will be submatriculating into the University of Pennsylvania School of Nursing Women's and Gender-Health Nurse Practitioner Program. *Our Hope for the Future,* Chapter 1, p. 19.

Linda MacIntyre, PhD, RN, PHN, FAAN, is Chief Nurse of the American Red Cross and provides oversight for Academic Service-Learning there, as well as being a HeartMath Master Trainer. *The American Red Cross: Volunteering in Times of Disasters,* Chapter 6, p. 109.

Jennifferre Mancillas, BSN, RN, RNC-NIC, is co-founder of the Lumify app, a Johnson & Johnson Nurse Innovation Fellow, and founder of the Community of Nurse Entrepreneurs. *The Benefits of Nurse-Led Innovation and the Barriers to Overcome,* Chapter 7, p. 136.

Donna J. Mazyck, MS, RN, LCPC, NCSN, CAE, FNASN, is Executive Director of the National Association of School Nurses. *The School Nurses' Collaborative Role in Health Equity for Students,* Chapter 5, p. 95.

Linda A. McCauley, PhD, RN, FAAN, FAAOHN, is Dean of the Nell Hodgson Woodruff School of Nursing at Emory University. *The Unexpected Power (and Joy) of Cross-Sector Collaborations*, Chapter 5, p. 87.

Derrick T. McCoy, Jr., BSN, RN, is a registered nurse at Grady Hospital. *Mentoring to Diversify*, Chapter 3, p. 50.

Donna Meyer, MSN, RN, ANEF, FAADN, FAAN, is CEO of the Organization for Associate Degree Nursing and an executive leader in the National Education Progression in Nursing Collaborative. *Achieving Health Equity Through Academic Progression*, Chapter 2, p. 32.

Rear Admiral Aisha K. Mix, DNP, MPH, RN, NHDP-BC, is Chief Nurse Officer in the US Public Health Service Commissioned Corps and represents HHS to the World Health Assembly, where she advises on nursing practice, education, and leadership as part of International Council of Nurses Government Chief Nurse and Midwifery Officers. *Leveraging Disaster Recovery for Community Preparedness*, Chapter 6, p. 112.

Adrianna Nava, PhD, MPA, MSN, RN, is President of the National Association of Hispanic Nurses and a research scientist with the Performance Measures Group at the National Committee for Quality Assurance. *The Voice of Advocacy: If Not You, Then Who?*, Chapter 10, p. 200.

Carolyn Nganga-Good, DrPH, RN, CPH, is Branch Chief at the Health Resources and Services Administration Bureau of Health Workforce in the Division of Practitioner Data Bank, where she oversees the Policy and Dispute Branch and is also a HeartMath Resilience Advantage Trainer. *Nurses as Champions for Bridging the Health Equity Gap*, Chapter 1, p. 16.

Adriana Perez, PhD, CRNP, ANP-BC, FAAN, FGSA, is Assistant Professor and Senior Fellow at the Leonard Davis Institute of Health Economics at the University of Pennsylvania School of Nursing, a scientist at the Center for Improving Care Delivery for the Aging, Penn's Resource Center for Minority Aging Research, and a board-certified adult nurse practitioner at Mercy LIFE. *Commitment to Advancing Health Equity With Hispanic/Latinx Communities Through Multi-Sector Collaboration*, Chapter 5, p. 92.

Elizabeth M. Perpetua, DNP, RN, ACNP-BC, ANP-BC, ARNP, FACC, is founder of Empath Health Services LLC, lecturer for the University of Washington School of Nursing Department of Biobehavioral Health and Informatics, and Adjunct Professor of Nursing at Seattle Pacific University. *Empowering Nurses to Own Our Pivotal Role in Advancing Technology, Innovation, and Entrepreneurship for Health Equity and Healthcare Transformation*, Chapter 7, p. 132.

Charlene Grace Platon, MS, RN, FNP-BC, is Director of Ambulatory Nursing at Stanford Health Care and CEO & co-founder of Fifth Window, a nurse-led and women-led digital wellness hub that matches nurses with self-care activities and resources and provides a supportive nursing community. *Crossing the Cultural Chasm Between Mental Health Stigma and Care-Seeking Behaviors in Nursing*, Chapter 8, p. 157.

Dame Anne Marie Rafferty, DPhil (Oxon), FAAN, FRCN, is Professor of Nursing Policy and Florence Nightingale Faculty of Nursing, Midwifery & Palliative Care at King's College London and Visiting Professor at the NIHR-funded Patient Safety Translational Research Centre, Imperial Healthcare NHS Trust. *Addressing the Worldwide Nursing Workforce Shortage: "There's no justice . . . just us"*, Chapter 9, p. 178.

Nacole Riccaboni, MSN, APRN, AGAC-NP, is a blogger and an advanced practice registered nurse in Florida, working on a Doctor of Nursing Practice degree at the University of Central Florida. *Voice of Nursing From the Front Lines*, Chapter 10, p. 193.

Cynda Hylton Rushton, PhD, RN, FAAN, is Anne and George L. Bunting Professor of Clinical Ethics at the Johns Hopkins Berman Institute of Bioethics and the School of Nursing, Chief Synergy Strategist for Maryland's R³ Resilient Nurses Initiative, co-chairs the Johns Hopkins Hospital's Ethics Committee and Consultation Service, and is editor and author of *Moral Resilience: Transforming Moral Suffering in Healthcare. Restoring Respect, Compassion, and Equity by Fostering Nurse Well-Being*, Chapter 8, p. 151.

Kathleen Sanford, DBA, RN, FAAN, FACHE, is Executive Vice President and Chief Nursing Officer for CommonSpirit Health. *Academia and Practice: Partnering for Diversity*, Chapter 3, p. 55.

Natalie Sanford, MSN, RN, is a PhD candidate at King's College London and King's Doctoral Student Association representative for the Florence Nightingale faculty of Nursing, Midwifery, and Palliative Care, where she also serves as the Research Executive PhD representative, chairs the faculty Journal Club, and teaches as a GTA and academic skills tutor. *Addressing the Worldwide Nursing Workforce Shortage: "There's no justice . . . just us"*, Chapter 9, p. 178.

Jewel Scott, PhD, RN, FNP-C, is a postdoctoral scholar at the University of Pittsburgh and serves on the Community Health Committee of Pittsburgh's Black Equity Coalition and the American Heart Association's Prevention Science Committee. *Health Equity and Black Maternal Mortality*, Chapter 1, p. 8.

Linda D. Scott, PhD, RN, NEA-BC, FNAP, FAAN, is Dean of the University of Wisconsin–Madison School of Nursing, President-Elect of the American Academy of Nursing, and Associate Editor for *Nursing Outlook*. *Progressing Beyond Holistic Admissions: Promoting Student Success to Transform the Nursing Workforce*, Chapter 2, p. 35.

Sarah L. Szanton, PhD, RN, FAAN, is Dean and Patricia M. Davidson Health Equity and Social Justice Endowed Professor at Johns Hopkins School of Nursing, holding joint appointments in the Department of Health Policy and Management at the Johns Hopkins Bloomberg School of Public Health and Johns Hopkins School of Medicine, core faculty at the Center on Aging and Health, the Hopkins Center for Health Disparities Solutions, and adjunct faculty with the Hopkins Center for Injury Research and Policy. *Addressing the Crack in the Healthcare Foundation*, Chapter 4, p. 74.

Carter Todd, MS, MBA, RN, CCRN, is Assistant Nurse Manager at Kaiser Roseville Medical Center and the current President and founder of the Capitol City Black Nurses Association. *Improving Healthcare by Meeting People Where They Are*, Chapter 4, p. 76.

Sylvia Trent-Adams, PhD, RN, FAAN, FNAP, is President at the University of North Texas Health Science Center at Fort Worth. Foreword, p. xxi.

Joanna Seltzer Uribe, EdD, MSN, RN, is currently a clinical nurse informaticist at the only female-owned hospital in New Jersey. *Nurses You Should Know: Inclusive Storytelling Designed to Expand the Nursing Narrative*, Chapter 10, p. 197.

Antonia M. Villarruel, PhD, RN, FAAN, is Margaret Bond Simon Dean of Nursing at the University of Pennsylvania School of Nursing, Director of the School's WHO Collaborating Center for Nursing and Midwifery Leadership, and serves as Co-Chair of the Strategic Advisory Council of the AARP/RWJ Future of Nursing: Campaign for Action. *Our Hope for the Future*, Chapter 1, p. 19.

Rachel (Rae) Walker, PhD, RN, is Associate Professor and Director of the PhD Program in the Elaine Marieb College of Nursing and Associate Director of the IALS Center for Personalized Health Monitoring at the University of Massachusetts Amherst. *Redistribute Power Over Data, Definitions, and Decision-Making*, Chapter 1, p. 12.

Jing Wang, PhD, MPH, RN, FAAN, is Dean and Professor of the Florida State University College of Nursing, Adjunct Professor in Biomedical Informatics and Public Health at the University of Texas Health Science Center at Houston, President of the Asian American/Pacific Islander Nurses Association, Editor-in-Chief of *JMIR Aging*, and Senior Policy Advisor for the Office of the National Coordinator for Health Information Technology and Centers for Medicare & Medicaid Services. *Diversity in Mentorship and Sponsorship for Nursing Leadership Development*, Chapter 3, p. 48.

Jill White, PhD, MHPol, MEd, RN, RM, is Professor Emerita of the Susan Wakil School of Nursing and Midwifery at the University of Sydney and Professor Emerita of the University of Technology Sydney, and is now an independent consultant in the areas of health education, regulation, and policy. *Global Stewardship: Reimagining the Adage "Think Global, Act Local" in the Post-Pandemic World—Every Nurse's Business*, Chapter 9, p. 181.

Maureen T. White, MBA, RN, NEA-BC, FNAP, FAAN, is Executive Vice President, Chief Nurse Executive for Northwell Health, Director of the Northwell Health Institute for Nursing, and Vice Dean for Health System Nursing Services at the Hofstra Northwell School of Graduate Nursing and Physician Assistant Studies. *Self-Care Is Not Selfish*, Chapter 8, p. 160.

Colonel Hope Williamson-Younce, DNP, ACNP-BC, CCNS, CEN, is Deputy Corps Chief for the US Army Nurse Corps, Office of the US Army Surgeon General, Defense Health Headquarters. *Learning Lessons From COVID-19: Upstream Fishing to Mend Downstream Implications*, Chapter 6, p. 122.

Launette Woolforde, EdD, DNP, RN, NPD-BC, NEA-BC, FAAN, is Chief Nursing Officer for Lenox Hill Hospital and the Manhattan region of Northwell Health and a Fellow of the New York Academy of Medicine and the American Academy of Nursing. *Self-Care Is Not Selfish*, Chapter 8, p. 160.

Tad Worku, RN, FNP-BC, is a songwriter, singer, speaker, and nurse practitioner. *Love Remains*, p. 147; *Peace of Mind*, p. 163; *Thirty3*, p. 184; *Won't Give Up*, p. 204.

Johnathan Zhu is an undergraduate BSN student at the University of Pennsylvania School of Nursing and an assistant for the Penn Nursing Innovation Department, where he has worked on initiatives such as Design Thinking for Health, the *Amplify Nursing* podcast, and the Penn Nursing Innovation Accelerator. *Innovation Approaches to Increasing Equity and Decreasing Harm*, Chapter 7, p. 143.

Deborah T. Zimmermann, DNP, RN, NEA-BC, FAAN, is Chief Executive Officer for the DAISY Foundation, President of the American Organization for Nursing Leadership, and a Fellow of the American Academy of Nursing. *Finding Our Voice of Advocacy*, Chapter 10, p. 190.

Table of Contents

Foreword

Over the past 50 years, there have been many advances in science, technology, and healthcare, but not everyone has benefited from these advances. Underserved and underrepresented groups have historically experienced significant disparities. The continued growth in health inequities cannot continue to be ignored. We know some things are not working, and change is needed to improve health and healthcare, especially for marginalized populations.

Taking Action: Top 10 Priorities to Promote Health Equity and Well-Being in Nursing is a timely discourse on the importance of nursing in addressing health equity and the complex structures and systems that drive inequities in healthcare. The authors explore how nurses can work to reduce health disparities, promote equity, and address structural racism.

Nurses have a critical role to play in achieving the goal of health equity and addressing structural racism, but they need robust education, supportive work environments, and autonomy. Nursing is well positioned to provide leadership in health equity and to build models of inclusion that allow providers, communities, and policymakers to come together to design actionable solutions.

This book explores the possibilities of creating pathways to empower nurses to be leaders in our communities and across the healthcare profession in the US and globally. It highlights the importance of bringing individuals together in a way that differences can be respected and serve as a catalyst for collaboration. Nurses are innovative and entrepreneurial. The profession is uniquely positioned to bring new technology, design thinking, and developments to healthcare to improve disparities and health equity.

The nursing profession can be a pivotal agent for change that promotes teaching, practice, advocacy, and collaboration in an environment of involvement, respect, and connection. It is critical that we find ways to identify shared ideas, backgrounds, and perspectives that create mutual benefit regardless of our social, political, or demographic differences. Nurses must demonstrate a sensitivity to and understanding of diverse populations and cultures to provide high-quality care across settings.

To overcome health equity challenges, there must be commitment from leadership at all levels of the healthcare system to promote diversity and inclusion as a part of the business model. Collaboration across all healthcare professions is key in developing an interprofessional team approach that puts the patient first, embracing cultural and social needs as well as physical and mental-health needs.

Taking Action presents a comprehensive discussion on the importance of global stewardship for the nursing profession. It also proposes a multisector approach to strengthen healthcare systems and the voice of nursing globally. This transformational book brilliantly outlines a vast array of inequities in health and opportunities for innovation and novel solutions.

–Rear Admiral (Ret.) Sylvia Trent-Adams, PhD, RN, FAAN, FNAP
Executive Vice President and Chief Strategy Officer
University of North Texas Health Science Center at Fort Worth

Preface

Nursing's Role in Advancing Health Equity

As the worst of the pandemic recedes in the United States, we have an opportunity to take stock of the past two years and imagine a brighter future. The pandemic has been devastating for far too many Americans who did not enjoy the luxury of being able to work from home, lacked access to healthcare, lived in crowded spaces, relied on public transportation, and have not gotten vaccinated. The elderly, people of color, and those who live in rural areas have been disproportionately affected by the pandemic in terms of illness and death (Iyanda et al., 2022). Over 1 million people in the US—a once inconceivable number— have died from COVID-19. More than 200,000 children have lost a parent or caregiver to COVID-19, and the shutdowns and school closures have unleashed a parallel mental health and educational crisis among youth (Leeb et al., 2020). In short, the pandemic exposed long-existing health disparities in our country that have persisted for generations. The nursing field is also hurting. Many nurses who have cared for an unrelenting stream of patients with COVID-19 are burned out, exhausted, and leaving the profession (Auerbach et al., 2022).

What happened is unacceptable, and our country must do everything in its power to dismantle health inequities and promote well-being for all. The nursing profession has tremendous potential to advance health equity, and we must commit to making health equity our North Star. We are the most trusted profession and the first contact for the majority of people who seek healthcare. We are bridge builders and collaborators who connect with people, communities, and organizations to improve health and well-being, and we are well positioned to combat the many shortcomings of the US health system (Pittman, 2019). Taking Action: Nurses' Role in Addressing Health Equity & Well-Being for All offers insight and advice from some of nursing's top minds about how we can unleash the potential of nurses to advance health equity. The authors, comprised of established and emerging leaders in public health, school nursing, health systems, and community settings, represent the diversity that we aspire to achieve in our profession. Achieving a more diverse workforce will ensure that our workforce reflects the US population and enable us to do a better job of providing culturally relevant care and eliminating persistent health disparities.

The contributors' wisdom reflects their expertise and lived experiences in advancing health equity, and their ideas mirror the recommendations set forth in the landmark report *The Future of Nursing 2020–2030: Charting a Path to Achieve Health Equity* (National Academies of Sciences, Engineering, and Medicine, 2021). This report, released in May 2021 during the pandemic and sponsored by the Robert Wood Johnson Foundation, calls for the systems that educate, pay, and employ nurses to permanently remove barriers to allow them to do this work, value their contributions, prepare nurses to tackle and understand health equity, and diversify the profession. The report emphasizes that nurse well-being is paramount to advancing the recommendations.

The good news is that the nursing field is ready to take on an expanded role in advancing health equity. Our profession has spent the past decade building its capacity to transform the healthcare system by implementing the recommendations from the then-named Institute of Medicine report, *The Future of Nursing: Leading Change, Advancing Health* (Shalala et al., 2011). The nursing field and our many partners, led by the Future of Nursing: Campaign for Action, a nationwide initiative of AARP, the AARP Foundation, and the Robert Wood Johnson Foundation, have strengthened nursing education, advanced practice, improved workforce diversity, and promoted nursing leadership. Together, we built the capacity of the nursing workforce to expand high-quality care to more Americans. But no one profession can advance health equity alone. Nurses need to join or form multi-sector partnerships with stakeholders from within and outside of healthcare, including educators, social justice organizations, community groups, consumer organizations, faith-based organizations, advocacy groups, health systems, broader community partners, and populations who have been disproportionately affected by the pandemic.

This decade, as we climb out of the ashes of the pandemic, the nursing field must set its sights on advancing health equity using the blueprint from the second future of nursing report to guide us. *The Future of Nursing: Campaign for Action* will work to catalyze the nursing field and our many partners to advance the report recommendations. Coalitions in nearly every state are developing strategic plans. To join them, go to www.campaignforaction.org and select "Get Involved."

There are many other ways for nurses to get involved. Nursing leaders can work to ensure that all nurses are able to practice to the full extent of their education and training. They can advocate for value-based payment reforms that better recognize and promote care coordination and transitional care. Nursing leaders can partner with schools of nursing to set up more clinical placements in the community. They can prioritize programs that promote nurse well-being, and they can serve as role models of well-being. They can keep abreast of what is happening on the front lines by spending time on floors and pitching in when necessary. Nursing leaders can form or join multi-sector partnerships and mentor and sponsor nurses from historically excluded backgrounds. They can set up seamless systems to screen for patients' needs and then partner with services that can help to meet those needs.

Nursing educators can develop competencies to advance health equity, initiate dialogues in their classrooms about racism and inequities, and mentor and sponsor students from historically excluded backgrounds in nursing. Deans and directors can create policies and regulations to protect students most at risk for behavioral health challenges, including students who may be experiencing economic hardships or feel they are unsafe, isolated, or targets of bias, discrimination, and injustice. They can ensure that all students can engage in virtual learning. Deans and directors can identify and eliminate policies, procedures, curricular content, and clinical experiences that perpetuate structural racism, cultural racism, and discrimination among faculty, staff, and students. They can recruit and put systems in place to support diverse faculty with expertise in the social determinants of health, population health, and health equity, and offer trainings to develop the skills of current faculty in these areas. Deans and directors can also build a more diverse pipeline by collaborating with local elementary and high schools to expose students to nursing as a career.

Frontline nurses can get involved in advancing health equity by modeling behaviors to promote diversity, equity, and inclusion on their floors. They can view themselves as leaders and develop innovations to improve care. They might engage in their communities to understand their strengths and assets. They can advocate for adding an assessment tool that can systematically collect data on a patient's social needs in the electronic health record. Frontline nurses can also advocate for themselves and others in the workplace, be effective team players, and develop coping and self-care skills.

Students can also play a role, from modeling behaviors that promote a culture of diversity, equity, and inclusion to getting involved in advocacy. Students can become aware of their own implicit biases and take trainings to address them, invest in their health, and identify and disseminate best practices to promote equitable care. Students can also seek out volunteer opportunities with organizations that are addressing the social determinants of health. They can also consider getting a PhD and conducting research to build the evidence base for advancing health equity.

The next decade offers tremendous challenges and opportunities for the nursing profession. More than ever, we need to tap the full potential of all nurses in every setting so that we can achieve what our county needs: for everyone—no matter who they are or where they live—to be able to experience good health and well-being. My hope is that *Taking Action: Top 10 Priorities to Promote Health Equity and Well-Being in Nursing* will inspire you to advance health equity.

                                                                    –Susan B. Hassmiller

References

Auerbach, D. I., Buerhaus, P. I., Donelan, K., & Staiger, D. O. (2022, April 13). A worrisome drop in the number of young nurses. *HealthAffairs*. https://www.healthaffairs.org/do/10.1377/forefront.20220412.311784/

Iyanda, A. E., Boakye, K. A., Lu, Y., & Oppong, J. R. (2022). Racial/ethnic heterogeneity and rural-urban disparity of COVID-19 case fatality ratio in the USA: A negative binomial and GIS-based analysis. *Journal of Racial and Ethnic Health Disparities, 9*, 708–721. https://doi.org/10.1007/s40615-021-01006-7

Leeb, R. T., Bitsko, R. H., Radhakrishnan, L., Martinez, P., Njai, R., & Holland, K. M. (2020, November 13). Mental health–related emergency department visits among children aged <18 years during the COVID-19 pandemic—United States, January 1–October 17, 2020. Centers for Disease Control and Prevention. *Morbidity & Mortality Weekly Report, 69*(45), 1675–1680. doi: 10.15585/mmwr.mm6945a3

National Academies of Sciences, Engineering, and Medicine. (2021). *The future of nursing 2020–2030: Charting a path to achieve health equity.* National Academies Press. https://www.nationalacademies.org/our-work/the-future-of-nursing-2020-2030

Pittman, P. (2019, March 12). *Activating nursing to address the unmet needs of the 21st century: Background paper for the NAM Committee on Nursing 2030.* Robert Wood Johnson Foundation. https://publichealth.gwu.edu/sites/default/files/downloads/HPM/Activating%20Nursing%20To%20Address%20Unmet%20Needs%20In%20The%2021st%20Century.pdf

Shalala, D., Bolton, L. B., Bleich, M. R., Brennan, T. A., Campbell, R., & Devlin, L. (2011). *The future of nursing: Leading change, advancing health.* National Academies Press. https://www.nap.edu/catalog/12956/the-future-of-nursing-leading-change-advancing-health

Introduction

Welcome to *Taking Action: Top 10 Priorities to Promote Health Equity and Well-Being in Nursing*. This book serves as the third edition of *The Power of Ten* (2011). So much has changed since the second edition (2017), including a major global pandemic, racial unrest with subsequent calls to address health equity and structural racism, and unanticipated nursing shortages that have affected the entire well-being of our profession. We based the top 10 issues highlighted in this book on the most relevant issues facing the nursing profession, as well as the people that nurses care for. Importantly, the second future of nursing report, *The Future of Nursing, 2020–2030: Charting a Path to Achieve Health Equity*, was released from the National Academies of Sciences, Engineering, and Medicine in May of 2021, thus providing an additional framework for the topics. Those issues or themes include:

1. Health equity

2. Education reform

3. Diversity and mentorship

4. Care delivery: quality, safety, access

5. Multi-sector collaboration

6. Preparing for disasters and public health emergencies

7. Innovation and entrepreneurship

8. Nurse well-being: compassion for self and others

9. Global stewardship

10. Nursing's voice in leading change

Similar to the second edition, we chose senior leaders well-versed in their chosen topics to contribute their expertise. With attention to diversity at all levels, including race, geography, gender, age, and sexual orientation, we asked the senior leaders to work with a mentee when possible to gain the perspective of up-and-coming leaders. Some of the essays were authored solely by up-and-coming diverse leaders, some of whom have never before published. To provide perspectives for all of nursing, we wanted all of nursing to be represented, or as much as we could for this small book. To gain such a diverse array of perspectives (66 essays in all), we limited each author to around 1,000 words. We have also supplemented the essays with notable quotes from experienced and novice leaders, in addition to the poetry and illustrations of **Lucinda Canty** and the song lyrics of **Tad Worku**.

We asked all authors to provide their essays based on evidence but also, importantly, their own lived experience. Due to the conversational tone of the essays, different writing styles will be encountered. Additionally, although we have not given any preference to particular nursing associations, some writers do come from associations, thus representing the work therein. Here is an overview of our top 10 issues and their contributors.

1 Health Equity

Nurses have a key role to play in addressing health equity on the front lines and beyond. Paying attention to these concepts and their application can improve health outcomes for all. **Ernest Grant**, President of the American Nurses Association, explains what is needed to dismantle structural racism, while frontline nurse practitioner **Whitney Fear**, a member of the Ogalala Sioux Tribe, states why it matters to build social capital in nursing with more intention than is currently given. **Jewel Scott**, a nurse scientist, provides suggestions for advancing health equity in Black mothers and pregnant women, and **Rachel Walker** and her colleague **Favorite Iradukunda** at the University of Massachusetts Amherst make the case that achieving health equity is a function of how it is defined and by whom. HRSA nurse administrator **Carolyn Nganga-Good** provides a rich example of how the COVID-19 pandemic has highlighted disparities, and the University of Pennsylvania School of Nursing Dean, **Antonia Villarruel**, and her student **Melina Lopez** plead that as nurses we must no longer remain silent to the injustices that lie before us and move to action. Indeed, it is our duty to take action, even if the solutions do not come overnight.

2 Education Reform

Kupiri Ackerman-Barger, an Associate Dean for Health Equity, Diversity, and Inclusion, maintains that the next generation of equity-minded nurses will need a unique knowledge base, skills, sense of self, and a bias toward collective efficacy. **David Benton**, CEO of the National Council of State Boards of Nursing, states that regulation, education, and services will all need to collaborate to design a fully articulate pathway to equip practitioners with the competencies needed to address health equity. **Donna Meyer**, CEO of the Organization for Associate Degree Nursing, believes that it is imperative that academic progression with community college graduates be strengthened to have the most highly educated and diverse nursing workforce. University of Wisconsin-Madison Dean, **Linda Scott**, supports the notion that approaching the student experience as a holistic process aimed at developing the breadth of nurses, while maintaining their own wellness needs, will produce a workforce better positioned to achieve health equity. Assistant Professor **Regina Eddie**, a member of the (Diné) Navajo Nation of Arizona and a voice for American Indian students, states that what is needed is a learning environment that embraces and improves a better understanding of American Indian students, their cultural background, and the influence of culture on life and learning experiences, attitudes, and beliefs.

3 Diversity and Mentorship

Wallena Gould, Founder and CEO of the Diversity in Nurse Anesthesia Mentorship program, presents a list of specific actions to help remove barriers to increase the number of diverse nurse anesthetists. Dean of Florida State University **Jing Wang** describes her strategies to increase diversity including a partnership with the Boys and Girls Club, which provides academic support and programming for first generation and underserved populations. **Derrick McCoy**, a Black male nurse at Grady Memorial, pays tribute to the mentors who helped him with his nursing career. Chief Diversity, Equity and Inclusion Officer at the American Association of Colleges of Nursing, **Vernell DeWitty**, asserts that although the percentage of graduates from nursing schools has increased by 10% from 2012–2022, it is still not representative of the general population. Executive Vice-President and Chief Nursing Officer of CommonSpirit, **Kathleen Sanford**, states that academia and practice must partner in implementing concrete strategies to increase the diversity of nurses and describes her attempts to do so. Duke Assistant Dean of the PhD program, **Rosa Gonzalez-Guarda**, claims that anti-racist frameworks are needed in nursing education that call for policies and actions that directly call out and address overt or covert manifestations of racism. **Gaurdia Banister**, Executive Director of the Institute for Patient Care at Massachusetts General Hospital, describes her beginnings as the only Black nursing student at her school and how she has started programs at her institutions to help bring more supportive strategies for nurses of color.

4 Care Delivery: Quality, Safety, Access

Cyrus Batheja and **Treyce Gladney**, leaders at UnitedHealthcare, describe how their company is now intentionally screening their members for social barriers, including the programs and resources in place to address those barriers. Chief Operating Officer at the Institute for Healthcare Improvement, **Cynthia Barginere**, portrays her personal journey correcting poor maternal morbidity and mortality rates for women of color and how she is now proudly serving at an institution dedicated to improving quality for maternal health. Johns Hopkins School of Nursing Dean, **Sarah Szanton**, describes a program she co-developed called CAPABLE: a participant-directed, home-based program that increases mobility and function of older adults in their home environment and decreases emergency department visits. **Julius Jonson**, an academician at the School of Nursing at Long Island University Brooklyn, and **Carter Todd**, an Assistant Nurse Manager at Kaiser Permanente, depict unique but familiar and comfortable locations to provide Black men's healthcare, including barber shops, the Black church, and nightclubs. **Billy Caceres**, Assistant Professor at Columbia University School of Nursing, provides his recommendations for nursing practice, research, education, and policy in an effort to improve care delivery for marginalized populations.

Multi-Sector Collaboration

Dean **Linda McCauley** of the Emory University Nell Hodgson Woodruff School of Nursing depicts how cross-disciplinary and cross-sector collaboration are essential in solving the complex issues of health inequity. Vice President of State Government Affairs for the American Association of Nurse Practitioners, **Tay Kopanos**, provides a vivid case study of how a failed effort with a piece of legislation was later rectified when a strong unified collaboration was formed. **Adriana Perez**, Associate Professor at the University of Pennsylvania School of Nursing, outlines challenges and strategies for multi-sector collaboration. Keys to collaboration include developing a shared agenda, clearly defining roles, finding funding and managing resources, and sharing data, says **Donna Mazyck**, Executive Director of the National Association of School Nurses. **Garrett Chan**, President and CEO of HealthImpact, explains how his company created VaxForce, a workforce management system to vet healthcare professionals and students and match them with existing vaccination events in partnership with community-based organizations. **Lauran Hardin**, Vice President and Senior Advisor for National Healthcare & Housing Advisors, highlights the need for creating community structures that allow for competitors to collaborate in a meaningful way.

Preparing for Disasters and Public Health Emergencies

The Chief Nurse of the American Red Cross, **Linda McIntyre**, describes how nurses can and should volunteer for her organization and the training needed to do so, while **Aisha Mix**, Chief Nurse of the Public Health Service, provides a comprehensive overview of how disasters affect health inequities. **Kathryn Booth**, Manager of Emergency Medical Services at Illinois Masonic Medical Center, illustrates how nurses serving in disasters and public health emergencies are victims themselves of stress and chaos and offers a methodology called HeartMath® as a resilience-building strategy. **Zenobia Harris**, nurse and Past President of the Association of Public Health Nurses, provides a historical overview of the pandemics that have plagued us and the need for a strengthened public health nursing sector. **Hope Williamson-Younce**, Deputy Corps Chief of the United States Army Nurse Corps, describes how the military provided support during the COVID-19 pandemic, within the context of achieving health equity.

Innovation and Entrepreneurship

Shawna Butler, a Healthtech Specialist and podcast host of *See You Now*, describes how COVID-19 accelerated the adoption of new technology but also revealed how easy it was to leave behind people without digital access, literacy, or devices—and the nurse's role in helping to correct this. **Liz Perpetua**, Founder and Chief Clinical Officer of Empath Health Services

LLC, calls nurses to action as natural innovators in the quest to achieve health equity, while **Jennifferre Mancillas,** Co-Founder and Chief Operating Officer of Lumify, encourages nurses to challenge the status quo within healthcare by keeping a forward-thinking mindset and by encouraging each other with nurse-led innovations. Program Director for Nursing Informatics at New York-Presbyterian Center for Professional Nursing Practice and Corporate Nursing and Filipino immigrant, **Mary Joy Garcia-Dia,** reports a clear lack of diversity in engaging with diverse populations during the technology development phase, which is leading to downstream health disparities and mistrust in technology. **Marion Leary,** Director of Innovation at the University of Pennsylvania School of Nursing, and her student, **Jonathan Zhu,** offer a variety of frameworks to achieve health equity through technology including human-centered design, equity-centered design, and Liberatory design, all underlined by Design Justice.

Nurse Well-Being: Compassion for Self and Others

Cynda Rushton, the Anne and George L. Bunting Professor of Clinical Ethics at the Johns Hopkins Berman Institute of Bioethics and the School of Nursing, calls for the active cultivation of more compassion for the very nurses who are called to deliver such. An action framework called G.R.A.C.E. is offered as the scaffolding for application. **Martha Dawson,** President of the National Black Nurses Association and Associate Professor at the University of Alabama at Birmingham, calls the nursing profession to action to have brave and curious action-oriented conversations to address racism and asks her white colleagues to become active allies, open to listening and learning. The Director of Ambulatory Nursing at Stanford Health Care and CEO and Co-Founder of Fifth Window, Filipino **Charlene Platon,** calls for the prioritization of addressing nursing mental health needs, while understanding the stigma that exists serving as a major barrier to care-seeking behaviors. **Maureen White,** Executive Vice President & Chief Nursing Executive at Northwell Health, and **Launette Woolforde,** Chief Nursing Officer at Lenox Hill Hospital, Northwell Health, outline what employers can and should do to promote nurse self-care, while describing their own strategies.

Global Stewardship

Yvonne Commodore-Mensah, Associate Professor at the Johns Hopkins School of Nursing, believes that all nurses are well positioned to advance health equity and improve health locally and globally, while particularly calling out high-income countries to collaborate globally with low- and medium-income countries to help them advance their scope of practice, training opportunities, research, and clinical practice. The current President of the International Council of Nurses and Dean at the University of Virginia School of Nursing, **Pam Cipriano,** believes nurses around the world must learn from each other and posts four case studies to help readers identify global strategies for providing access to care for marginalized populations. Three leaders at the Pan American Health Organization, including **Silvia Cassiani**, **Bruna Moreno Dias**, and **Cashimro Canha Cavaco Dias**, and their colleague from the Ministry of Health and Wellness of Jamaica, **Patricia Ingram-Martin**, all pay testament to nurses' leadership during the COVID-19 pandemic but claim that to be prepared for the future, a much greater investment in resources must be made within the nursing profession. **Anne Marie Rafferty**, Professor of Nursing Policy at King's College London, and her PhD student, **Natalie Sanford**, believe that nurses must intervene at every level by building on the United Nations Commission on Employment and Economy as well as the World Health Organization Assembly resolution on nursing and midwifery, using these recommendations as nursing's calling card to hold governments accountable and translate these into tangible strategic goals to influence policy. Professor Emerita of the Susan Wakil School of Nursing and Midwifery University of Sydney, **Jill White**, states there is nothing a nurse does that does not have consequences, ultimately for their patients, the community, the country, and the planet—from waste reduction to voting with knowledge and consciousness to actively collaborating on evidence to improve practice. It all matters.

Nursing's Voice in Leading Change

Paule Joseph, the Lasker Clinical Research Scholar at the National Institutes of Health, strongly expresses the need for nurses to examine, unpack, and mitigate their own biases and dismantle the policies and structures that hold inequity in place. **Deborah Zimmermann**, CEO of the Daisy Foundation and President of the American Organization of Nurse Leaders, believes that the disruption caused by the pandemic has provided a great window of opportunity for all nurses to convene, educate, advocate, and innovate to become active strategists to lead our countries to better health. School nurse and Clinical Coordinator at Rutgers University, **Robin Cogen**, describes how she raised awareness and concerns that school nurses were facing through her popular blog, *The Relentless School Nurse*, now read by over 300,000 people. **Ravenne Aponte**, a PhD student at the University of Pennsylvania School of Nursing, and **Joanna Seltzer**, a Johnson & Johnson Innovation Fellow, shined the light on their online learning platform, "Nurses You Should Know," which was created to diversify the nursing narrative by conveying stories of past and present-day nurses of color through bite-sized videos and blogs. And **Adriana Nava**, President of the National Association of Hispanic Nurses, tells of her own leadership journey with many times being the only Latina in the room to a current position of national prominence, where her mission is to lead other Hispanic nurses to policy and other leadership-oriented fields.

Reference

National Academies of Sciences, Engineering, and Medicine. (2021). *The future of nursing 2020–2030: Charting a path to achieve health equity.* National Academies Press. https://nam.edu/publications/the-future-of-nursing-2020-2030

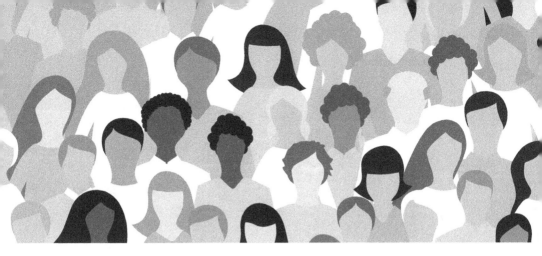

1 Health Equity

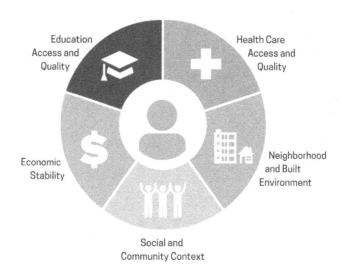

Figure 1.1   Social determinants of health.
(US Department of Health and Human Services & Office of Disease Prevention and Health Promotion, n.d.)

This chapter focuses on the nurse's role in promoting health equity on the front lines and beyond, providing equitable care, addressing social determinants of health (see Figure 1.1), and dismantling structural racism. Social determinants of health lead to disparate health outcomes, but as nurses, it is imperative that we move beyond this acknowledgment and take action to promote equitable healthcare services so that everyone receives care that optimizes their health. When we recognize that a person's cultural and social backgrounds affect where, when, how, and if they receive healthcare services, it is no longer acceptable to uphold a system that provides the same care for every patient (equality). Instead, a system that takes an individual's needs into account to create a personalized plan of care (equity) should be endorsed. A shift toward health equity is a shift toward improved healthcare outcomes for all.

Consider the following questions as you read the essays about health equity:

- Why should nurses care about health equity?

- What are some examples of how biases and stereotypes held by nurses negatively affect health equity and health outcomes?

- What roles can nurses play in bridging the health equity gap across healthcare and in the community?

- What actions can nurses take to dismantle structural racism and improve health equity?

- What are some local, state, and national resources and organizations available to support the nurses' journey toward health equity?

This Is a Journey: Dismantling Structural Racism

Ernest J. Grant, PhD, DSc(h), RN, FAAN
ANA President

Nursing today has been forced to recognize that racism does exist within the profession, with the patients we care for and in the world around us. Surveys conducted by the National Commission to Address Racism in Nursing only confirm what we already knew (Singer, 2022). In addition, the pandemic has also exacerbated and shone a light on healthcare disparities and racism. This is something that members of the BIPOC (Black and Indigenous people of color) community knew existed all along. But how do we tear down those walls so that everyone can be seen for who they are and the contribution that they make to society versus the opposite? What can I, as a nurse, and my fellow nurse colleagues do to ensure racism is no longer tolerated in nursing, in healthcare, and in society? The answer is very complex. We know that racism is a public health crisis that impacts mental, spiritual, and physical health. We know that racism can make individuals and the communities in which they live feel undervalued, unappreciated, and not cared for. One has only to look at communities of color in any town or city and note the vast differences in available resources as compared to the more affluent side of town.

"Of all the forms of inequality, injustice in healthcare is the most shocking and inhumane."

–Dr. Martin Luther King, Jr.
Civil Rights movement leader

As nurses we need to continue to address the need for respect, equity, inclusion, and social justice within healthcare and within the nursing profession. We must also speak up to our colleagues when we see acts of racism occurring, such as the "zip code test" serving as a proxy for race in a residentially segregated US to predict outcomes, or the "wallet test" to determine whether a comprehensive workup may be performed (Alcalde, 2018; UC Santa Cruz, n.d.). Other things that nurses can do to begin to dismantle racism include:

- **Using your individual voice and influence** to educate others about systemic injustices, health inequities, and health disparities. Instead of "going along with the group" to maintain peace, I challenge nurses to be disrupters and call out racism and discrimination when they encounter it. You are adhering to the Code of Ethics, which obligates all nurses to be allies and to speak up against racism, discrimination, and injustice (American Nurses Association, 2015).

- **Educating yourself** and then using your trusted voice and influence to educate others about the systemic injustices that continue to be perpetuated throughout healthcare and society at large. It is important that nurses first understand and comprehend how structural racism presents itself. In healthcare, sometimes it's in the way students are educated or perhaps a poorly written textbook that mistakenly draws conclusions about ethnic groups. Think of the modern eugenics movement that swept through the US in the early 20th century, leading to laws prohibiting miscegenation and the forced sterilization of undesirable "races" in an effort to create a better, more intelligent, whiter nation (Bailey et al., 2021).

- **Being aware of your own unconscious bias.** Essentially, *unconscious biases* are the results of our own personal experiences and societal interactions that may influence our thoughts and actions without us knowing it (Long, 2015). It is important that nurses first recognize that they can be biased, and once they realize it, begin to work on ways to eliminate this issue. A great way to begin chipping away at unconscious biases is to practice a simple approach such as questioning yourself about your thoughts, comments, etc.; developing a sense of core values; being inclusive of others; and setting an example for others to follow. This is not something that can be changed overnight, but the first step is to recognize that we all have biases, and it's how we present or channel those biases that may determine whether we hold ourselves accountable.

- **Standing up for inequity and calling it what it is.** Perhaps one of the most difficult things for an individual to do is to confront a colleague or superior when it comes to inequity. The fact that it could result in retaliation, charges of insubordination, loss of career advancement, or job loss is always looming when such attempts are made and may cause an individual to pause before acting. However, doing what is right and just should be your guiding principle, as it will make everyone in the workplace environment feel a sense of well-being and belonging. Becoming an ally and speaking in a manner that is thoughtful, measured, and non-threatening is one way to call out inequity and the least likely way to cause colleagues to react defensively.

Finally, as nurses we must be committed to implementing comprehensive strategies to address inequities and dismantle structural racism. We must continue to take action and advocate on behalf of those who are made to endure acts of racism in its many forms. Yes, I still have to keep reminding myself that this is a journey—a very long journey on which there is still much work to be done. I hope that you will join me on this journey to ensure that the nursing profession is representative of everyone and the people that we serve!

References

Alcalde, M. G. (2018, Nov. 29). Zip codes don't kill people—Racism does. *HealthAffairs*. https://doi.org/10.1377/forefront.20181127.606916

American Nurses Association. (2015). *Code of ethics for nurses with interpretive statements* (2nd ed.). Author. https://www.nursingworld.org/coe-view-only

Bailey, Z. D., Feldman, J. M., & Basset, M. T. (2021). How structural racism works—Racist policies as a root cause of U.S. racial health inequities. *New England Journal of Medicine, 384*(8), 768–773. https://www.nejm.org/doi/10.1056/NEJMms2025396

Long, K. (2015, December 14). How to recognise and overcome your unconscious bias. *The Guardian*. https://www.theguardian.com/women-in-leadership/2015/dec/14/recognise-overcome-unconscious-bias

Singer, A. (2022). National survey of nurses finds extensive racism in the workplace. *Campaign for Action*. https://campaignforaction.org/survey-finds-extensive-racism-nursing/

UC Santa Cruz. (n.d.). *Tool: Recognizing microaggressions and the messages they send*. https://academicaffairs.ucsc.edu/events/documents/Microaggressions_Examples_Arial_2014_11_12.pdf

US Department of Health and Human Services & Office of Disease Prevention and Health Promotion. (n.d.). *Healthy People 2030. Social determinants of health*. https://health.gov/healthypeople/priority-areas/social-determinants-health

Building Social Capital in Nursing: Doing With Intention

Whitney Fear, MSN, PMHNP-BC
Psychiatric Mental Health Nurse Practitioner
Family Healthcare

As research has expanded on the social determinants of health, so too has the volume of conversations about how to best address the extent of the inequities revealed by the study of this topic. The potential for these conversations to result in the just changes needed to decrease health inequity is entirely dependent on the quality of these discussions and whether those with inherent privilege are willing to acknowledge the ways in which that privilege has either directly or indirectly contributed to the continuance of health disparities. Nursing has an opportunity to address inequity, both within our profession and for our patients, through a willingness to experience the discomfort of the vulnerability that is required for the development of truly meaningful interventions.

> *"Nursing is a dynamic field that requires courage. Courage to stand on the side of the people we serve. Courage to partner with communities to design and test interventions. Courage to lead. I am really grateful that I get to be a part of that nursing future because I believe that fear only works on those who are afraid, and I walk with courageous people."*
>
> –Monica McLemore, PhD, MPH, RN, FAAN
> Professor, Department of Child, Family, and
> Population Health Nursing
> University of Washington, School of Nursing

Often, minoritized groups are seen only for how at-risk they are and not often enough for what they could be offering our profession in the way of knowledge and building resilience within communities. A *maǎké* (sister friend) of mine once remarked to me, "Something that is so fascinating to me about native people is that everything that you do has a purpose and a reason for doing it." This is true. We don't do small talk. We don't create meaningless processes. We believe that every word we speak and every action that we take should be done with intention. I believe that the least meaningful interventions for reducing systemic barriers in healthcare have come from shrinking goals to the micro level for precision. In that process, the intention often shifts to creating a goal that is satisfactory by the standards of science and no longer focused on the original intention of correcting an injustice. An example is the creation of loan repayment programs as a solution for diversifying the nursing workforce. That appears to be a solution that makes sense when considering financial barriers of accessing an education. However, it totally misses the mark as far as considering that many of the students who would use those loan repayment programs won't even be able to gain admission to nursing school. Many of us grow up in areas where even the best students can't access the classes required for admission to nursing school because they aren't offered. Those super precise solutions disregard the fact that the education system in the US is exclusionary of diverse people, and the education offered to disadvantaged populations is often of a lower quality. Perhaps, instead, the solution should be to remove the systemic discrimination embedded in the education system rather than continuing to subject diverse persons to the injustice of that systemic discrimination.

The only rule that I have for colleagues and acquaintances about participating in conversations about my own personal experiences with systemic barriers and the discrimination that I feel is present in healthcare, based on observations as a nurse, is that they first contemplate if they are truly ready for that. If diverse people are expected to extend ourselves emotionally to help our colleagues understand the breadth of discrimination that exists throughout the continuum of healthcare, then our colleagues had better be ready to listen. I'd like to clarify what I mean by listening, which is that our colleagues ought to come to those conversations ready to overcome their own impulses to become defensive when confronted with the reality of how the same systems that they benefit from are simultaneously, dangerously, and fatally oppressing millions of others so that they are ready to work with us on formulating solutions.

It takes vulnerability for us to extend ourselves in the way that is required to share those experiences. When much of your life has involved a struggle and met opposition for the most basic of resources, one of the last things you want to do is show another person your fracture points. If someone has ever shared those types of things with you, they have ignored a very strong impulse to protect themselves because they have hope that you will do something positive with that information. Please read that again and try to think of all the times that a patient or their loved one has shared a story of experiencing discrimination, racism, sexism, etc., with you and realize the weight of the opportunity that was presented to you in that moment. If you are without an example in mind, this is most likely because you have not presented yourself as someone deserving of that level of trust, and it would serve you (and your patients) well to perform some introspection about why that would be.

I want to acknowledge that it takes courage to begin to examine how the structure of our society has afforded us an advantage that has not been afforded to another. This is a point in which it is tempting to instead name all the adversity that you have experienced, yet that is not productive during a conversation about the oppression of a population to which you do not belong. Rather than using these openings to respond by explaining all the difficulties in life that you have had or throwing out examples of people who have "pulled themselves up by their bootstraps," these moments can be used to build social capital.

What is social capital? *Social capital* refers to the connections among people in society that offer resources and support. When we create relationships with people who are from different backgrounds, we create bridging social capital. Connecting ourselves or helping to link others to individuals/organizations of influence creates linking social capital. Mutual trust and investment in those connections are completely necessary for those increases in social capital that result from bridging and linking (Berner et al., 2020).

Increased social capital is associated with lower rates of crime, higher rates of academic achievement, and healthier individuals/families (Berner et al., 2020). Nurses are in a unique position to help build both bridging and linking social capital. I encourage nurses to think about how nurses can help to build social capital that would improve the overall well-being of all people and the areas within nursing that lack those connections that we see demonstrated as a lack of diversity within our profession.

Reference

Berner, M., Brown-Graham, A., Mills, B., Graham, P. W., Landwehr, J., Lawrence, S., Benton, A., Erickson, L., & Martinez, S. (2020). *The value of relationships: Improving human services participant outcomes through social capital.* US Department of Health and Human Services. https://aspe.hhs.gov/sites/default/files/migrated_legacy_files//196286/SocialCapital-Handbook-Sept-2020.pdf

Health Equity and Black Maternal Mortality

Jewel Scott, PhD, RN, FNP-C
Assistant Professor, University of South Carolina College of Nursing

Black women in the United States have a greater likelihood of perinatal death than any other racial or ethnic group (Bond et al., 2021). So, while overall maternal mortality in the US is abysmal, for Black mothers and birthing people, the mortality rate ratio (maternal deaths per 100,000 births) is 37.1, more than double that of white and Hispanic women in the US (Bond et al., 2021). In discussing health equity and maternal mortality, it is critical to acknowledge the historical and contemporary racism at the core of the disparities in mortality, as described in *Medical Apartheid* (Washington, 2006).

> "To create a more humane healthcare system by fostering health equity and justice for populations of color, organized nursing must eliminate racism from its own structural systems by becoming more socially just, diverse, equitable, and inclusive."
>
> —Freida Hopkins Outlaw, PhD, RN, APRN, FAAN
> Executive Program Consultant, American Nurses Association

Combatting the alarming Black maternal mortality crisis will require an intentional effort from all healthcare professionals, including nurses. A critical and equitable approach to resolving the Black maternal mortality crisis is to "center on the margins." That means identifying the "extreme cases" or the population(s) overrepresented among maternal deaths and designing tailored, focused interventions in collaboration with community-based organizations and community members. Interventions that occur at the neighborhood or population level and focus on the extremes may yield improvements for all or at least a leveling of the playing field. My nursing practice and emerging research have focused on the margins to illuminate the challenges and collaborate with the community to identify solutions.

As a family nurse practitioner, I have had the privilege to provide prenatal care at several federally qualified health centers, which provide care to the medically marginalized (e.g., those with no health insurance). Due to the social stratification of society and the US employment-based health insurance system, most of my patients were Black and Latinx females. Often, they expressed appreciation for having a Black healthcare provider, and my training as a nurse and experience with trauma-related research informed my philosophy of caring for the whole person. I imagine that it may have helped that we shared some similar life experiences.

Representation matters in all settings, and research findings suggest better outcomes when patients-providers are race concordant, although results are mixed (LaVeist & Nuru-Jeter, 2002; Sacks, 2018). However, none of the studies reviewed in a 2009 systematic review were conducted in obstetric settings (Meghani et al., 2009). A more recent study identified that race-concordant patient-provider matches reduced infant mortality, especially in the case of medically complex infants (Greenwood et al., 2020). Provider-patient race concordance is an area for future research, as many believe that increasing racial/ethnic diversity in nursing and healthcare will resolve the problem. It will help, but it is important to remember that racism in the US is a groundwater problem where absorbing many of the same images and veiled messages can result in internalized racism among Black individuals, as described in *A Gardner's Tale* (Jones, 2020).

I also practiced in less traditional settings, most recently with Healthy Start, a federally supported home visiting program, to implement the Centering Group Prenatal Care model in response to the racial disparities in severe maternal morbidity and mortality in Pittsburgh (Healthy Start, 2022). Working with a community-based organization reverses the common healthcare approach of expecting patients to come to us. Home visiting programs are one evidence-based tool for reducing and eliminating racial disparities in maternal mortality. Other high-income countries with significantly lower maternal mortality ratios employ nurses to visit every mom/birthing parent at their home in the days and weeks after delivery (Health Resources Services Administration, 2021; Tikkanen et al., 2020). Considering that nearly 20% of postpartum deaths occur in the first six days at home, having a trained nurse in the home in that critical period could reduce maternal deaths (Tikkanen et al., 2020).

The following suggestions are specific to the role of nurses in advancing health equity for Black mothers and pregnant people:

- It is essential for nurses to become more self-aware of their implicit biases. In addition to taking implicit association tests, nurses are encouraged to pause when deciding on care for a patient and ask how bias might be working, similar to the timeout procedures used in operating rooms. Nurses may need support to develop a reflexive practice. One example is adding guided reflections to students' assignments to stimulate the critical self-appraisal needed to identify biases (Johnson & Richard-Eaglin, 2020).

- Of the approximately 40 nurse-midwifery programs in the US, zero are at the 15-plus nursing schools at Historically Black Colleges and Universities. As acknowledged earlier, diversifying the workforce is not the only solution, but it is impossible to overstate that representation matters and the importance of diversity. Many of the regulations governing midwifery were passed at a time when higher education was largely inaccessible for Black people, creating an area of nursing that continues to be 90% white (Suarez, 2020; Tobbell, 2021).

- Expanded nurse-led home visiting partnerships and other innovations are also action items that could promote health equity. Cardiovascular disease is the number one preventable cause of maternal death (Bond et al., 2021). In the perinatal period, trained nurses providing additional education, support, and blood pressure assessments could identify problems sooner. Black women are over-represented in the 5–10% of women who develop preeclampsia, and there are few evidence-based interventions, and none tailored for the women at the margins (Jowell et al., 2021).

- Nursing must evaluate whether the current policy and advocacy training provided to nurses across the continuum is effective. With the passing of H.R. 1318, Preventing Maternal Deaths Act, maternal mortality review committees are now present in all states. However, there is little guidance on the makeup of the committees, and not much information is available on the disciplines represented and the demographic makeup of the review committees (Kozhimannil et al., 2019). This is just one example of how nursing can be more engaged in policy to advocate for patients, who are better served when nurses have a voice in policy decisions.

This list will hopefully generate new thoughts, conversation, and, most importantly, action; I encourage readers to see other articles that focus on how nursing can respond to emerging and long-standing inequities more broadly (Johnson et al., 2020; Scott et al., 2020).

References

Bond, R. M., Gaither, K., Nasser, S. A., Albert, M. A., Ferdinand, K. C., Njoroge, J. N., Parapid, B., Hayes, S. N., Pegus, C., Sogade, B., Grodzinsky, A., Watson, K. E., McCullough, C. A., & Ofili, E. (2021). Working Agenda for Black Mothers: A position paper from the Association of Black Cardiologists on Solutions to Improving Black Maternal Health. *Circulation: Cardiovascular Quality and Outcomes, 14*(2), e007643. https://doi.org/10.1161/circoutcomes.120.007643

Greenwood, B. N., Hardeman, R. R., Huang, L., & Sojourner, A. (2020). Physician–patient racial concordance and disparities in birthing mortality for newborns. *Proceedings of the National Academy of Sciences, 117*(35), 21194–21200. https://doi.org/10.1073/pnas.1913405117

Health Resources Services Administration. (2021). *The maternal, infant, and early childhood home visiting program*. https://mchb.hrsa.gov/sites/default/files/mchb/about-us/program-brief.pdf

Healthy Start. (2022). *Healthy communities, healthy families, healthy babies, healthy start*. https://healthystartpittsburgh.org/

Johnson, R., & Richard-Eaglin, A. (2020). Combining SOAP notes with guided reflection to address implicit bias in health care. *Journal of Nursing Education, 59*(1), 59. https://doi.org/10.3928/01484834-20191223-16

Johnson, R., Scott, J., & Randolph, S. D. (2020). COVID-19 and Black America: The intersection of health equity and the NP workforce. *The Nurse Practitioner, 45*(10), 11–14. https://doi.org/10.1097/01.NPR.0000696932.97210.37

Jones, C. P. (2000). Levels of racism: A theoretic framework and a gardener's tale. *American Journal of Public Health, 90*(8), 1212. https://doi.org/10.2105/ajph.90.8.1212

Jowell, A. R., Sarma, A. A., Gulati, M., Michos, E. D., Vaught, A. J., Natarajan, P., Powe, C. E., & Honigberg, M. C. (2021). Interventions to mitigate risk of cardiovascular disease after adverse pregnancy outcomes: A review. *JAMA Cardiology, 7*(3), 346–355. https://doi.org/10.1001/jamacardio.2021.4391

Kozhimannil, K. B., Hernandez, E., Mendez, D. D., & Chapple-McGruder, T. (2019). Beyond the Preventing Maternal Deaths Act: Implementation and further policy change. *HealthAffairs*. https://www.healthaffairs.org/do/10.1377/hblog20190130.914004/full/

LaVeist, T. A., & Nuru-Jeter, A. (2002). Is doctor-patient race concordance associated with greater satisfaction with care? *Journal of Health and Social Behavior, 43*(3), 296–306.

Meghani, S. H., Brooks, J. M., Gipson-Jones, T., Waite, R., Whitfield-Harris, L., & Deatrick, J. A. (2009). Patient–provider race-concordance: Does it matter in improving minority patients' health outcomes? *Ethnicity & Health, 14*(1), 107–130. https://doi.org/10.1080/13557850802227031

Sacks, T. K. (2018). *Invisible visits: Black middle-class women in the American healthcare system*. Oxford University Press.

Scott, J., Johnson, R., & Ibemere, S. (2020). Addressing health inequities re-illuminated by the COVID-19 pandemic: How can nursing respond? *Nursing Forum, 56*(1), 217–221. https://doi.org/10.1111/nuf.12509

Suarez, A. (2020). Black midwifery in the United States: Past, present, and future. *Sociology Compass, 14*(11), 1–12. https://doi.org/10.1111/soc4.12829

Tikkanen, R., Gunja, M., FitzGerald, M., & Zephrin, L. (2020). *Maternal mortality and maternity care in the United States compared to 10 other developed countries*. The Commonwealth Fund. https://www.commonwealthfund.org/publications/issue-briefs/2020/nov/maternal-mortality-maternity-care-us-compared-10-countries#32

Tobbell, D. (2021). *Black midwifery's complex history*. University of Virginia School of Nursing. https://www.nursing.virginia.edu/news/bhm-black-midwives/

Washington, H. A. (2006). *Medical apartheid: The dark history of medical experimentation on Black Americans from colonial times to the present*. Doubleday Books.

Redistribute Power Over Data, Definitions, and Decision-Making

Rachel (Rae) Walker, PhD, RN, FAAN
Associate Professor and PhD Program Director, Elaine Marieb College of Nursing
University of Massachusetts Amherst

Favorite Iradukunda, PhD, RN
Assistant Professor, Elaine Marieb College of Nursing
University of Massachusetts Amherst

Healthcare is increasingly dominated by calls for data-driven decision-making (National Academies of Science, Engineering, and Medicine, 2021). Every day, nurses generate data that are archived and shared through platforms like electronic health records. Although most do not identify as informaticists or data scientists, numbering more than 27.9 million globally, nurses represent one of the largest contingents of data workers in the world (World Health Organization, 2020).

Big data and artificial intelligence (AI) have been framed as imperatives for the future of health and care (Ronquillo et al., 2021). We are also seeing more discussions about data ethics, including the importance of addressing data bias (Obermeyer et al., 2021). What most conversations omit, however, is a critical analysis of power, how power operates to shape data, and the possibilities created (or precluded) by the worlds those data create.

"I was surprised when at the end of a recent hospital stay, a nurse came to my room and announced she needed to educate me on smoking cessation. I'd never smoked, but she was adamant, implying my chart said so. This worried me—how had such clearly false information gotten there, and what else might be inaccurate? How would these errors further impact my care as a Black woman? She minimized my concerns. The data in my file spoke far louder than my voice."

–Favorite Iradukunda

Whether or not we achieve health equity is a function of how it is defined and by whom. Such decisions reflect arrangements of power. Health equity is not achievable when what it is and how to get there remain defined and operationalized exclusively by those who possess unearned advantages under current regimes. Co-creating new futures where health equity is even a possibility, much less a universal reality, will require fundamentally redistributing power over definitions, data, and decision-making.

As members of a self-described "caring profession," nurses use data to heal and promote health. But caring by itself is not enough, as all data can be weaponized to further marginalize and harm those we work with and for (Benjamin, 2019). This is especially true when data are generated and applied without accountability to those impacted. Nurse leaders must be prepared to reckon with the origins, narratives, and power behind data, to implement accountability practices, and to engage in acts of repair where harm has already occurred (Johnson, 2021). Data practices should be constantly and critically analyzed through the lens of power, including how data are structured, generated, analyzed, archived, presented, and shared.

Data storytelling, especially acts of "talking about, without," entails myriad threats to health equity such as deficit models. *Deficit models* involve norming data to dominating groups (like cisgender white settlers), while othering anyone who falls outside such norms, defining them in terms of deficiencies and pathology (Bryant et al., 2021). Deficit models are foundational to much of the health disparities discourse (Rabelais & Walker, 2021). By focusing on "disparity," without naming the structures that created it (e.g., settler colonialism, cisheteropatriarchy, or white supremacy), deficit models shape narratives that place the burden of reform entirely on those being harmed, reifying existing oppressions.

Nurses should also be reflexive about data hierarchies, wherein certain ways of knowing—like the use of numbers, statistics, or big data—are given greater legitimacy than practices that cede narrative control to communities. Data that are quantitative, easy to access, or "machine-learning ready" are far more likely to be used in decision-making, even when they reinforce, rather than challenge, the status quo (Gebru, 2022).

Data feminism calls us to embrace multiple ways of knowing, including moving beyond static and artificially "objective" data displays toward elevating emotion and embodiment in data, a practice actively discouraged under current data regimes (D'Ignazio & Klein, 2020). Glitching—a cyberfeminist practice of refusal—rejects artificial binaries and hegemonic data models like electronic health records, treating places where data refuse to "fit" the model not as errors but as opportunities for emancipatory practice (Russell, 2020).

We must make visible the invisible labor and resources underpinning big data and its management. Much of this labor is performed by minoritized persons who are under-waged or unpaid (Crawford & Joler, 2018). Resource demands include extractive and environmentally racist supply chains required to power data-driven technologies like AI and the blockchain, and their staggering carbon costs (Hao, 2019).

Data have a life beyond their creation. A power lens interrogates archival practices, asking questions like:

- Do communities impacted have control over the life (or destruction) of the data, after its initial purpose has been fulfilled?

- Who decides what gets shared, with whom, and under what circumstances and systems of accountability?

- Whose comfort and priorities are being centered?

Health equity is not possible under current regimes of power. But we must try to create new futures, even when results fall far short of the ideal. To paraphrase Dr. Monica McLemore's model of reimagine, retrofit, and reform, we can't all be on team utopia (McLemore, 2021). Navigating data practices with integrity requires curiosity, humility, reflexivity, accountability, recognition of our mutual interdependence, and reckoning with racism and other oppressions; a willingness to engage in refusal where necessary (Cifor et al., 2019); and grief work to acknowledge stories we have told ourselves and internalized (that were never true) and harm caused by those stories and the worlds they've built. Which also means that we need repair practices and—in the recent words of AI ethics leaders like Timnit Gebru and Jenny L. Davis—*algorithmic reparations* that place resources and power directly in the hands of marginalized communities (Davis et al., 2021; Gebru, 2022).

We've often heard that data do not—*cannot*—"speak for themselves." The unspoken corollary is that stories told with data are products of human choices. Data storytelling by dominating groups should never trump the voices and agency of persons marginalized under current power regimes. What health equity is and how it is measured are data questions, bound up in power. Justice in the realm of data, definitions, and decision-making is an exercise in accountability around the redistribution of power.

References

Benjamin, R. (2019). *Race after technology: Abolitionist tools for the New Jim Code*. Polity.

Bryant, J., Bolt, R., Botfield, J. R., Martin, K., Doyle, M., Murphy, D., Graham, S., Newman, C. E., Bell, S., Treloar, C., Browne, A. J., & Aggleton, P. (2021). Beyond deficit: 'Strengths-based approaches' in indigenous health research. *Sociology of Health & Illness, 43*(6), 1405–1421. https://doi.org/10.1111/1467-9566.13311

Cifor, M., Garcia, P., Cohen, T., Rault, J., Sutherland, T., Chan, A., Rhode, J., Hoffman, A., Salehi, A., & Nakamura, L. (2019). *Feminist data manifest-No*. https://www.manifestno.com

Crawford, K., & Joler, V. (2018, September 7). *Anatomy of an AI system*. AI Now Institute and Share Lab. http://www.anatomyof.ai

Davis, J. L., Williams, A., & Yang, M. W. (2021). *Algorithmic reparation*. Big Data & Society. https://doi.org/10.1177/20539517211044808

D'Ignazio, C., & Klein, L. F. (2020). *Data feminism*. MIT Press.

Gebru, T. (2022, March 22). *The hierarchy of knowledge in machine learning and its consequences*. ADVANCE Distinguished Lecture, University of Massachusetts Amherst. https://www.umass.edu/advance/events/hierarchy-knowledge-machine-learning-and-its-consequences-advance-distinguished-lecture-dr

Hao, K. (2019, June 6). Training a single AI model can emit as much carbon as five cars in their lifetimes. *MIT Technology Review*. https://www.technologyreview.com/2019/06/06/239031/training-a-single-ai-model-can-emit-as-much-carbon-as-five-cars-in-their-lifetimes/

Johnson, K. (2021, December 23). A move for "algorithmic reparation" calls for racial justice in AI. *WIRED*. https://www.wired.com/story/move-algorithmic-reparation-calls-racial-justice-ai/

McLemore, M. (2021). *The role of Title X and TPP in maternal morbidity and mortality prevention*. Reproductive Health National Training Center. https://rhntc.org/sites/default/files/resources/supplemental/rhntc_role_title_x_tpp_maternal_transcript_5-18-2021.pdf

National Academies of Science, Engineering, and Medicine. (2021). *The future of nursing 2020–2030: Charting a path to achieve health equity*. National Academies Press. https://nam.edu/publications/the-future-of-nursing-2020-2030/

Obermeyer, Z., Nissan, R., Stern, M., Eaneff, S., Bembeneck, E. J., & Mullainathan, S. (2021). *Algorithmic bias playbook*. Center for Applied AI at Chicago Booth.

Rabelais, E., & Walker, R. K. (2021). Ethics, health disparities, and discourses in oncology nursing's research: If we know the problems, why are we asking the wrong questions? *Journal of Clinical Nursing, 30*(5–6), 892–899. https://doi.org/10.1111/jocn.15569

Ronquillo, C. E., Peltonen, L.-M., Pruinelli, L., Chu, C. H., Bakken, S., Beduschi, A., Cato, K., Hardiker, N., Junger, A., Michalowski, M., Nyrup, R., Rahimi, S., Reed, D. N., Salakoski, T., Salanterä, S., Walton, N., Weber, P., Wiegand, T., & Topaz, M. (2021). Artificial intelligence in nursing: Priorities and opportunities from an international invitational think-tank of the Nursing and Artificial Intelligence Leadership Collaborative. *Journal of Advanced Nursing, 77*(9), 3707–3717. https://doi.org/10.1111/jan.14855

Russell, L. (2020). *Glitch feminism: A manifesto*. Verso.

World Health Organization. (2020, April 6). *State of the world's nursing 2020: Investing in education, jobs and leadership*. https://www.who.int/publications-detail-redirect/9789240003279

Nurses as Champions for Bridging the Health Equity Gap

Carolyn Nganga-Good, DrPH, RN, CPH
Health Resources and Services Administration Administrator

Nurses are well-positioned to promote health equity and address social and structural determinants of health (SSODH). Health equity means that everyone has what they need to have the best possible health outcomes. Nurses in frontline settings such as health departments, schools, correctional facilities, primary care centers, and emergency departments (EDs) work at the healthcare entry point for many people. They can play a crucial role in assessing and addressing SSODH. Nurses who work in academia, administration, policy, and legislation who also sit at decision-making tables have the opportunity to influence education, practice, policy, and funding decisions that address SSODH and health disparities and promote health equity.

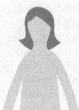

"There is no health equity without nurses, who represent half of the world's healthcare workforce. To improve health equity, invest in and empower nurses."

–Elizabeth Madigan, PhD, RN, FAAN
Chief Executive Officer, Sigma Theta Tau International

To achieve sustainable health equity, we must consider healthcare outside the four walls of healthcare facilities as people come from somewhere and return somewhere. Efforts within the healthcare system will be futile if there is no follow-up when the client returns home. As the most trusted profession, nurses have the opportunity to influence their clients' health outcomes by building a good rapport, assessing the client's living and work situations, identifying barriers, linking them to resources that help address those barriers, and providing health education. Coupled with care coordination and case management efforts, partnerships with community-based organizations (CBOs) can help address SSODH and promote health equity. Such an approach by hospitals, third-party payers, and CBOs has proved successful in managing chronic diseases. Utilizing paraprofessionals such as community health workers, patient advocates, and navigators has also proven to be effective in improving healthcare access and health outcomes. Successful strategies include emphasizing prevention, improving health literacy by educating clients on the importance of regular checkups and healthy living, and encouraging appropriate use of the healthcare system by focusing on primary care and urgent care instead of using the ED for their primary care needs.

Integrating health systems and providing comprehensive medical and social services in one-stop shops have been effective in helping clients access services, keeping them in care, and achieving better health outcomes, especially for marginalized populations. For example, an ED offered universal routine HIV testing to clients who had come to the ED for other health reasons. Newly diagnosed clients were immediately connected to an HIV provider and case manager; those who disclosed being previously diagnosed but had fallen out of care were reconnected to care while still in the ED. Barriers such as lack of housing, medical insurance, and transportation were assessed during that ED visit and subsequently addressed in future clinic visits. Structural barriers such as the proximity of the providers to reliable public transportation, clinic hours, and clinic co-payment policies were also considered. Clients were followed up in the community through a partnership between the hospital, local health department, community providers, and CBOs. These efforts improved HIV linkage to care, retention, and adherence (Menon et al., 2016).

Health systems can no longer work in silos if they want to optimize their performance, achieve health equity, and meet the Quadruple Aim—reduce health costs and improve patient experience, population health outcomes, and provider experience. These efforts cannot happen in a vacuum or without resources. Payment mechanisms to help address SSODH should be established and enhanced; this requires political will and intentionality to invest in efforts that improve health equity. For example, Maryland's all-payer model and global budgeting that requires both private and public payers to pay the same established rate for hospital services reduces payment disparities and incentivizes hospitals to better manage patients' health outcomes, reduce re-hospitalization, and appropriately manage chronic diseases outside the acute care setting (Health Services Cost Review Commission, 2018). However, caution should be taken to ensure that the quest to reduce costs doesn't exacerbate health inequalities due to unequal opportunities, barriers, and biases.

Implicit biases, unconscious biases, and stereotyping negatively impact health equity and health outcomes. Examples are common: a sickle cell patient being labeled as a drug seeker; someone living in a food desert with no access to fresh food and no reliable/affordable means of transportation being labeled as non-compliant for having uncontrolled blood pressure and diabetes; a homeless person being ordered medications they cannot afford and that require refrigeration and then being labeled as a frequent flyer when they keep getting readmitted to the hospital for the same conditions.

The COVID-19 pandemic has highlighted the disparities in our communities, including essential workers who did not have paid sick leave who we expected to stay home when they were sick; workers without insurance or the underinsured who frequently deferred care and only sought care when they were very sick, often in the ED; and working parents without paid parental leave who needed to place their young infants in commercial day cares, exposing them to frequent infections such as colds. It is critical to assess these structural barriers and the clients' living and working situations to identify and address barriers that may further impede the achievement of optimal health, including addressing mental health and substance use disorders.

Educators should not only teach nurses their role in improving health equity so that they are ready to apply it in their day-to-day work but also practice it with their students to ensure that the same SSDOH that affect their clients do not hold the students back from graduating and becoming the best providers they can be. Nurses can also be catalysts and innovators for best practices and strategies, providing equitable care, addressing SSDOH and disparities, and promoting individual and population health. In addition to advocating for equitable care for their patients and communities, nurses can play a critical role in formulating and improving policies and legislation to improve health equity.

In conclusion, addressing health equity requires a combined effort between policy, practice, and education. Nurses at all levels of practice and settings are uniquely placed to play critical roles in ensuring the provision of equitable care, addressing SSODH and disparities, and dismantling implicit biases, unconscious biases, and stereotypes. The time is now, the place is here, and each of us has a duty to promote health equity wherever we are.

References

Health Services Cost Review Commission. (2018, April). *Monitoring of Maryland's new all-payer model: Biannual report.* https://hscrc.maryland.gov/Documents/legal-legislative/reports/April%202018%20Biannual%20Report%20FINAL%20051118.pdf

Menon, A. A., Nganga-Good, C., Martis, M., Wicken, C., Lobner, K., Rothman, R. E., & Hsieh, Y. H. (2016). Linkage-to-care methods and rates in U.S. emergency department-based HIV testing programs: A systematic literature review brief report. *Academic Emergency Medicine, 23*(7), 835–842. https://doi.org/10.1111/acem.12987

Our Hope for the Future

Melina Lopez, BSN, RN
Graduate nurse, University of Pennsylvania

Antonia M. Villarruel, PhD, RN, FAAN
Professor and Margaret Bond Simon Dean of Nursing
University of Pennsylvania School of Nursing

From a global pandemic to supremacist terror, to issues regarding climate change and border control, to the possibility of a third world war, the promise of a near future is threatened. These past years have disrupted and shattered how we lived, learned, worked, and dreamt about our lives, families, goals, and careers. Instead, for many "normality" has been replaced by worries about the wake of another surge of COVID-19, exacerbated by rising misogynistic, racist, homophobic, and classist sentiments that govern our healthcare, our policies, our communities, and yes—even our profession. The political climate has raised fears about our very democracy, fueled by the January 6th insurrection, voter suppression, and lack of judicial justice. This has also called into question the ability to pursue our passions for health equity—including the health and well-being of racial and ethnic minoritized communities, immigrant health, LGBTQ health, and reproductive healthcare, specifically abortion and gender-affirming care.

Nursing organizations, schools, and healthcare systems have responded, especially after the killing of George Floyd, with statements and commitments to address structural racism. The close to 3 million nurses in the United States have a unique role in addressing structural and institutional factors that produce health inequities. But where to start?

First, we must start with a careful and critical examination of how the profession of nursing has been complicit in supporting structural racism. We must scrutinize and correct the virtuous image that is perpetuated about the origins of the nursing profession in general and specifically in the US. We need to amplify the history and the voices of nurses of color—as told by these nurses. This is an important reckoning if we are ever to lead in promoting health equity. We must not only diversify the nursing workforce but also ensure that racial and ethnic minoritized nurses are seen and heard and provided opportunities to lead within the profession.

We must invest in our future—our students—and support and prepare them to lead in achieving health equity. Students want and need to discuss current events in light of their personal and professional goals and responsibilities. As educators, we need to ensure that we make space for discussion of current events and their personal and professional impacts. Content and discussions about structural and social determinants of health—as well as levers for change at the personal, institutional, and societal level—should not be isolated to a class on cultural competence or cultural humility, or a course on social determinants, health policy, or ethics. They should be deliberately threaded throughout the entire nursing curriculum. We also need to include our clinical partners and preceptors as part of the conversation.

This investment in our students to advance health equity requires the ability to create and maintain a supportive environment for open and honest discussions. It also requires skills that educators may need support in developing. Importantly, it will take effort to "decolonize" the curriculum.

Finally, consistent with the American Nurses Association Code of Ethics (2015), we must be engaged in social justice to achieve health equity. This includes "analysis, critique and change of social structures, policies, laws, customs, power and privilege that disadvantage or harm vulnerable social groups through marginalization, exclusion, exploitation, and voicelessness" (p. 46). Nurses must use their individual and collective voices—wherever they live, work, play, and pray. We must use our respected status as the most trusted profession and no longer remain silent to the injustices we see. Importantly, we need to use our political power as a profession and as individuals to dismantle structures and processes that disadvantage others. It is important to recognize that our activism should not be limited to what others must do, but we must also be reflective and hold ourselves accountable to our actions and inaction.

We will not fix structural racism overnight, nor will we achieve health equity tomorrow. These efforts require a sustained commitment and a great deal of work from each of us. We may not get it right the first time. We may not always say or do the "right" thing. Let that not stop us from moving forward. Let us teach and support each other as we move forward. We must use the experiences of the past two years—as horrific as they have been—to propel us to a new way of leading and being.

Reference

American Nurses Association. (2015). *Code of ethics for nurses with interpretive statements*. Author. https://www.nursingworld.org/coe-view-only

My Profession, Nursing

Since I was a small child
I dreamed of being a nurse
White hat
White dress
White shoes

I wanted to care for those who couldn't care for themselves
To provide comfort when one's in pain
To provide hope when one's uncertain
To provide a listening ear when one is afraid to speak

I became a nurse before I knew who I was as a person
I cared for the most vulnerable before learning how to care for myself
Nursing became a profession I grew to love
Like a relationship with ups and downs
A relationship with several challenges
A relationship, I knew I would never leave

It was in nursing
Where I learned about myself
Where I found my voice
Where I understood my purpose
My desire to care for others strengthened
Erasing all thoughts of self-doubt
No longer questioning my right to be a nurse
No longer afraid, no longer silent
My Profession, Nursing

Poetry by Lucinda Canty, PhD, CNM, FACNM
Associate Professor of Nursing, University of Massachusetts Amherst

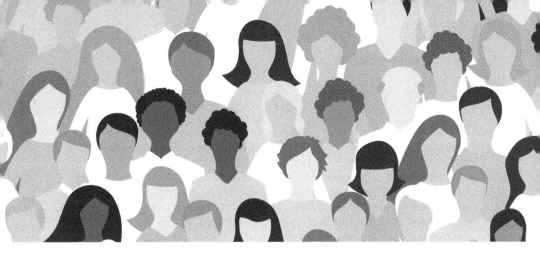

2 Education Reform

In This Chapter

- The Who, What, How, and When of Nursing Workforce Diversity

- Demographics, Diversity, Education, and Health Outcomes

- Achieving Health Equity Through Academic Progression

- Progressing Beyond Holistic Admissions: Promoting Student Success to Transform the Nursing Workforce

- A Tool to Promote Cultural Humility to Advance Academic Success for American Indian/Alaska Native Nursing Students

Education reform to promote health equity is discussed in this chapter. It is imperative that we understand what should be taught to advance nursing education to the point that it addresses harmful biases, eliminates discrimination in learning environments, and cultivates an inclusive environment (cultural humility). Furthermore, an emphasis on health equity must persist throughout all aspects of nursing education—from admissions to curriculum design to graduation. This approach is required for the nursing profession to truly embrace and exemplify the characteristics that align with improving health equity. Nursing education has the power to influence student nurses in unique ways that impact when, where, and how they care for others. Educating future nurses to practice through a health equity lens will undoubtedly lead to increased health equity and thus, improved health outcomes.

Consider the following questions as you read the essays about health equity and education reform:

- What are some ways in which schools of nursing can promote health equity?

- Describe/define the following terms: cognitive diversity, equity-minded, equity pedagogy, and cultural humility.

- What are the differences between the historical/traditional and holistic admission processes?

- What are some challenges to nursing school success for minoritized students?

- How does diversifying the nursing workforce through nursing education affect health equity?

The Who, What, How, and When of Nursing Workforce Diversity

Kupiri Ackerman-Barger, PhD, RN, CNE, ANEF, FAAN
Associate Dean for Health Equity, Diversity and Inclusion
University of California Davis Betty Irene Moore School of Nursing

The Value of Nursing Workforce Diversity— The Who

To appreciate the value of nursing workforce diversity, it is important to view diversity from several vantage points. When we think of diversity as a driver of excellence, we understand that ensuring diversity in the nursing workforce is more than "the right thing to do" but rather a necessity for providing high-quality equitable care across individuals, families, communities, social groups, and populations. Diversity brings an advantage to the power of thinking, problem-solving, and innovation. Page (2017) uses logic to emphasize the intellectual capacity of teams of people who interpret, reason, and problem-solve differently from each other, a concept known as *cognitive diversity*. Further, diverse and inclusive teams can generate inclusive and relevant research questions and enhance innovative approaches to solving complex healthcare issues (Swartz et al., 2019). Diversity among nursing researchers can broaden what is researched, how it is researched, and how those data are interpreted.

"The health equity movement is just that: a movement of people committed to advancing health equity for all communities. It requires the participation and unwavering commitment of all of us, working together to address the determinants of health and advocating for improving the quality of life for those who have been historically ignored and excluded from opportunities afforded other privileged groups."

–David R. Williams, PhD, MPH
Florence Sprague Norman and Laura Smart Norman Professor of Public Health
Chair of the Department of Social and Behavioral Sciences
Harvard T. H. Chan School of Public Health
Professor of African and African American Studies and Sociology, Harvard University

In addition to diverse thinkers, we need representation in all areas of nursing practice. In terms of patient care, a diverse and representative nursing workforce provides more opportunities for patients to receive healthcare from professionals who share similar identity traits. Evidence has shown that there is increased satisfaction and trust, as well as better communication within racially concordant healthcare interactions (Blanchard et al., 2007; Shen et al. 2018). Representation in nursing leadership is needed to inform institutional decision-making that creates and sustains equity. These decisions include, but are not limited to, hiring and promotion practices as well as ensuring that underheard voices are at the table during policy and resource allocation discussions. Representation is needed in nursing education where nursing knowledge and theories are constructed and disseminated; curricula is designed; topics are emphasized or omitted; and perspectives are included, stereotyped, or overlooked. Further, racially and identity concordant education can improve student satisfaction, give prospective and current students role models, and create an overall sense of belonging.

Equity-Minded Nurses—The What

The Future of Nursing 2020: Charting a Path to Achieve Health Equity report highlighted that nurses are well positioned to address health inequities and have "the potential to reshape the landscape of health equity" (National Academies of Sciences, Engineering and Medicine, 2021, p. 127). However, to do this, nurses need the knowledge, skills, and sense of self and collective efficacy to do so. A fundamental place to start is to focus on the upstream factors that impact health outcomes such as the social and political determinants of health (Dawes, 2020). Nurses often avoid engagement in politics because it is complex, messy, and rarely provides immediate gratification for one's efforts. However, to radically change disparate outcomes in healthcare we must collectively tackle the structures, policies, and laws that created them and perpetuate them. At four million strong, nurses are well poised to make the political impact needed to advance health equity, but to do so, we must be equity-minded.

The Center for Urban Education coined the term *equity-minded*. Using their definition and adapting it for nursing practice, we might say:

> Equity-minded nurses are those who are willing to assess their own racialized assumptions and recognize how these assumptions can impact their clinical decision-making, to acknowledge their lack of knowledge about the history of race and racism and how this history impacts current health outcomes, to take responsibility for optimizing the health and wellness of historically underserved and minoritized individual patients, communities and population, and to critically assess racialization in their own practices as nurses, educators, researchers and/or leaders. (McNair et al., 2020, p. 20)

As schools engage in curriculum reform to advance health equity, the mission should be to graduate nurses who are equity-minded. We need curricula that provides the social and political context for health outcomes (Ackerman-Barger et al., 2020). This approach, referred to by Chinn and Kramer (2008) as emancipatory knowing in nursing, is the "human ability to recognize social and political problems of injustice or inequity, to realize things could be different, and to piece together complex elements of experience and context in order to change a situation as it is, to a situation that improves people's lives" (p. 77).

Best and Promising Practices in Nursing Education—The How

In addition to what is taught, it is essential to transform the way we educate future nurses so that they enter nursing practice as equity-minded professionals. Banks (2016) discussed the notion of equity pedagogy in his multicultural education model. *Equity pedagogy* refers to teaching in such a way that maximizes opportunities for all learners to engage with the material and to be successful in their academic pursuits. Multi-model teaching and evaluation approaches are one way to provide numerous opportunities for learners to engage with the material and demonstrate what they know. Another way to practice equity pedagogy is through a deep commitment to creating and sustaining inclusive classroom environments where students from all backgrounds feel that their contributions and perspectives are valued and add to the overall learning in the classroom. Practicing cultural humility in nursing learning environments not only role models behavior that can translate into quality patient care but leverages the power of diversity through inclusion and a sense of belonging. *Cultural humility* describes a way of being that involves self-reflection, self-critique, and an active pursuit of lifelong learning (Tervalon & Murray-Garcia, 1998). For nurse educators, this means that we actively reframe the faculty-to-student power dynamic and interrogate our assumptions about what we think we know about individuals, families, and communities of people. We need to check our assumptions about students' capabilities, motivation, and roles as learners. Using a cultural humility framework, we assume that individuals from groups different from our own have the wisdom and the ability to teach and learn, to problem solve, and to innovate. It is the role of educators to create the kind of learning environment where students learn from each other and where teaching and learning are reciprocated between students and nurse educators.

Envisioning Our Future—The When

In nursing and in healthcare it is imperative for us to appraise our history, celebrate our successes, and rectify injustices. We need to understand how our legacy, discipline norms, and social and political structures inform our discipline and shape our current outcomes. This is not an exercise in self-flagellation, rather a realistic look at where we have been and where we are so that we can soberly chart a path to the future nursing and health outcomes that align with our values of social justice and health equity.

References

Ackerman-Barger, K., London, M., & White, D. (2020, November). When an omitted curriculum becomes a hidden curriculum: Let's teach to promote health equity. *Journal of the Healthcare for the Poor and Underserved, 34*(1), 182–192. https://doi.org/10.1353/hpu.2020.0149

Banks, J. A. (2016). *Cultural diversity and education: Foundations, curriculum, and teaching* (6th ed.). Routledge.

Blanchard, J., Nayar, S., & Lurie, N. (2007). Patient-provider and patient-staff racial concordance and perceptions of mistreatment in the health care setting. *Journal of General Internal Medicine, 22*(8), 1184–1189. https://doi.org/10.1007/s11606-007-0210-8

Chinn, P. L., & Kramer, M. K. (2008). *Integrated theory and knowledge development in nursing.* Mosby Elsevier.

Dawes, D. (2020). *The political determinants of health.* Johns Hopkins University Press.

McNair, T. B., Bensimon, E. M, and Malcolm-Piqueux, L. (2020). *From equity talk to equity walk: Expanding practitioner knowledge for racial justice in higher education.* Jossey-Bass.

National Academies of Sciences, Engineering and Medicine. (2021). *The future of nursing 2020–2030: Charting a path to achieve health equity.* The National Academies Press. https://doi.org/10.17226/25982

Page, S. (2017). *The diversity bonus: How great teams pay off in the knowledge economy.* Princeton University Press.

Shen, M. J., Peterson, E. B., Costas-Muñiz, R., Hernandez, M. H., Jewell, S. T., Matsoukas, K., & Bylund, C. L. (2018). The effects of race and racial concordance on patient-physician communication: A systematic review of the literature. *Journal of Racial and Ethnic Health Disparities, 5*(1), 117–140. https://doi.org/10.1007/s40615-017-0350-4

Swartz, T. H., Palermo, A. S., Masur, S. K., & Aberg, J. A. (2019). The science and value of diversity: Closing the gaps in our understanding of inclusion and diversity. *The Journal of Infectious Diseases, 220*(S2), S33–S41. https://doi.org/10.1093/infdis/jiz174

Tervalon, M., & Murray-Garcia, J. (1998). Cultural humility versus cultural competence: A critical distinction in defining physician training outcomes in multicultural education. *Journal of Healthcare for the Poor and Underserved, 9*(2), 117–125. https://doi.org/10.1353/hpu.2010.0233

Williams, D. (2020). Foreword. In D. Dawes, *The political determinants of health* (p. xi). Johns Hopkins University Press.

Demographics, Diversity, Education, and Health Outcomes

David C. Benton, PhD, RN, FRCN, FAAN
Chief Executive Officer, National Council of State Boards of Nursing

Despite spending by far the most on healthcare, as a percentage of its gross domestic product, the United States continues to be last in terms of health outcomes when compared with 10 similar high-income countries (Schneider et al., 2021). This is an enormous and pernicious topic that must be addressed if key indicators such as falling life expectancy, access to care, shortages of health practitioners, and inadequate diversity of the workforce are to be resolved.

It is not possible to provide a comprehensive solution set to all the problems that the US health and education systems face in this short essay, but instead a focus on changing demographics, the need for increased diversity of the workforce, and the opportunity to learn from others are considered.

Population Demographics: Increasing Percentage of Elderly and More Ethnic Diversity

Parker et al. (2019) identified that the number of older Americans as a percentage of the total population is increasing and that this will place additional burdens on the delivery of healthcare. The same authors also note that the composition of the population is set to become more racially and ethnically diverse (2019). This is not a surprise for demographics as the age and ethnic structure of the US has been changing dramatically since the 1950s. At that time there were 25 live births per 1,000 of the population, but today this number has dropped to 14, a number that is projected to decline further over the next 30 years (Congressional Research Service, 2011). Indeed, the US Census Bureau (2020) has noted that by 2060 nearly one in four Americans is projected to be an older adult. At the same time the Census Bureau projects that the population will become more ethnically diverse, as immigration will need to increase around the year 2030 to meet the increasing need for workers to provide services to older persons (2020).

From these stark facts it is important to conclude that the demand for nursing care will increase and the supply will become tighter as the dependency ratio will double between 2010 and 2060—i.e., currently there are 21 people aged 65 and older for every 100 in the workforce, but by 2060 there will be 41 (US Census Bureau, 2020). More positively, the diversity of the available workforce is likely to increase, but this may not match the profile of the population needing care as immigration will be the main driver of addressing workforce shortages.

Educational Landscape, Diversification Response, and Continuum of Practice

The US is no different from other nations with regard to the challenges of obtaining timely, comprehensive data on educational provision, employment, and deployment relating to the nursing workforce (World Health Organization, 2020). Nursing care is provided by a wide array of practitioners ranging from support workers to advanced practice nurses (International Council of Nurses, 2008). In the US, the education for such practitioners can be provided by employers, departments of health, community colleges, and the university sector, resulting in a highly fragmented array of provision.

It has been recognized that there is a mismatch between the ethnic profile of practitioners and the patients and populations they serve (Gilliss, 2010; Zangaro et al., 2018). Despite this recognition, little progress has been made in increasing the diversity of the non-white licensed nursing workforce with the LPNs fluctuating around 30% and RNs remaining fixed between 19.2 and 19.5% from 2015 until 2020 (Budden et al., 2016; Smiley et al., 2018, 2021). Furthermore, data on support workers illustrate that ethnic diversity is much higher in this group ranging from 63% for home care workers, 58% for nursing assistants to 52% for residential care aides (Paraprofessional Healthcare Institute, 2021). Clearly, with the use of articulated pathways, accreditation for prior learning and prior experiential learning coupled with career ladders and lattices, as used in other countries such as the United Kingdom, the potential to expand the diversity of the licensed nursing workforce already exists and is much needed if the demographic challenges ahead are to be met (Johnson et al., 2013; Triby, 2009; United Kingdom Central Council for Nursing, Midwifery and Health Visiting, 1999).

As noted above, the doubling of the dependency ratio will present significant challenges, and an all-graduate nursing workforce will not be possible nor appropriate, but if access to needed services is to be available for all, then all levels of practitioner will need to work to their full scopes of practice and limits of their education. Regulation, education, and services will all need to collaborate to redesign a fully articulated pathway that equips practitioners with the necessary competencies to meet healthcare needs and promote well-being if the current reduction in US life expectancy is to be reversed. Furthermore, lessons need to be learned from other countries that have expanded the scopes of practice of both the licensed practical nurse and the registered nurse. For example, in an increasing number of high- and low-income countries, registered nurses can prescribe, make referrals, and so much more, facilitating a more coherent, safe, and accessible service to all (International Council of Nurses, 2021; Kooienga & Wilkinson, 2017).

Conclusions

This essay has only scratched the surface of what is ahead of the profession. Multiple solutions to the problems facing education, service delivery, and redesign in the United States have already been solved by many other nations. Nurse leaders must have the foresight to consider these as opportunities, reject the mantra of ignoring what was not invented locally, and embrace with passion and confidence the potential to implement and improve solution sets that increase access to services and offer an education pathway that not only can lift individuals out of poverty but set them on a progressive career that will be in high demand as American society ages and modes of delivery evolve.

References

Budden, J. S., Moulton, P., Harper, K. J., Brunell, M. L., & Smiley, R. (2016). The 2015 National Nursing Workforce Survey. *Journal of Nursing Regulation Supplement, 7*(1), S1–S90. https://doi.org/10.1016/S2155-8256(16)31055-9

Congressional Research Service. (2011). *The changing demographic profile of the United States.* Author. https://sgp.fas.org/crs/misc/RL32701.pdf

Gilliss, C. (2010). Making the case for nursing workforce diversity. *Nursing Outlook, 58*(5), 223–224. https://doi.org/10.1016/j.outlook.2010.07.002

International Council of Nurses. (2008). *Nursing care continuum framework and competencies.* Author. https://siga-fsia.ch/files/user_upload/07_ICN_Nursing_Care_Continuum_Framework_and_Competencies.pdf

International Council of Nurses. (2021). *Guidelines on prescriptive authority for nurses.* Author. https://www.icn.ch/system/files/2021-09/ICN_Nurse_prescribing_guidelines_EN_WEB.pdf

Johnson, S., Scammell, J., & Serrant-Green, L. (2013). Degrees of success: Safeguarding an ethnically diverse nursing workforce in nursing education. *Journal of Psychological Issues in Organizational Culture, 3*(1), 321–345. https://doi.org/10.1002/jpoc.21069

Kooienga, S., & Wilkinson, J. (2017). RN prescribing: An expanded role for nursing. *Nursing Forum, 52*(1), 3–11. https://doi.org/10.1111/nuf.12159

Parker, K., Moring, R., & Horowitz, J. M. (2019). *Looking to the future, public sees an America in decline on many fronts.* Pew Research Center. https://www.pewresearch.org/social-trends/2019/03/21/public-sees-an-america-in-decline-on-many-fronts/

Paraprofessional Healthcare Institute. (2021). *Direct care workers in the United States: Key facts.* Author. https://phinational.org/wp-content/uploads/2021/09/Direct-Care-Workers-in-the-US-2021-PHI.pdf

Schneider, E. C., Shah, A., Doty, M. M., Tikkanen, R., Fields, K., & Williams II, R. D. (2021). *Mirror, mirror 21 – Reflecting poorly: Health care in the U.S. compared to other high-income countries.* The Commonwealth Fund. https://www.commonwealthfund.org/sites/default/files/2021-08/Schneider_Mirror_Mirror_2021.pdf

Smiley, R. A., Lauer, P., Bienemy, C., Berg, J. G., Shireman, E., Reneau, K. A., & Alexander, M. (2018). The 2017 National Nursing Workforce Survey. *Journal of Nursing Regulation, 9*(3), S1–S88. https://doi.org/10.1016/S2155-8256(18)30131-5

Smiley, R. A., Ruttinger, C., Oliveira, C. M., Hudson, L. R., Allgeyer, R., Reneau, K. A., Silvestre, J. H., & Alexander, M. (2021). The 2020 National Nursing Workforce Survey. *Journal of Nursing Regulation, 12*(1), S1–S90. https://doi.org/10.1016/S2155-8256(21)00027-2

Triby, E. (2009). Accreditation of prior experiential learning and the development of higher education. *European Journal of Vocational Training, 46*(1), 114–128. https://files.eric.ed.gov/fulltext/EJ864792.pdf

United Kingdom Central Council for Nursing, Midwifery and Health Visiting. (1999). *Fitness for practice: The UKCC Commission for Nursing and Midwifery Education*. United Kingdom Central Council.

US Census Bureau. (2020). *Demographic turning points for the United States: Population projections for 2020 to 2060*. Author. https://www.census.gov/content/dam/Census/library/publications/2020/demo/p25-1144.pdf

World Health Organization. (2020). *The State of The World Nursing Report 2020: Investing in education, jobs and leadership*. Author. https://apps.who.int/iris/rest/bitstreams/1274201/retrieve

Zangaro, G. A., Streeter, R., & Li, T. (2018). Trends in racial and ethnic demographics of the nursing workforce: 2000 to 2015. *Nursing Outlook, 66*(4), 365–371. https://doi.org/10.1016/j.outlook.2018.05.001

Achieving Health Equity Through Academic Progression

Donna Meyer, MSN, RN, ANEF, FAADN, FAAN
Chief Executive Officer, Organization for Associate Degree Nursing

It is hard to believe the Institute of Medicine's (IOM) landmark study, *The Future of Nursing: Leading Change, Advancing Health*, was published over 10 years ago (2010). Its release marked a pivotal time in our country as massive healthcare reform was enacted, population demographics were veering towards an aging and chronically ill society, and the delivery of healthcare was transitioning from acute care to a community-based care model. The report offered a blueprint for the future that reflected our nation's complex, evolving healthcare system and explained how nurses' roles, responsibilities, and education should adapt to meet the needs of an aging, chronically ill, and increasingly diverse population. The eight recommendations outlined in the IOM report aimed to improve healthcare for all Americans by enhancing nurses' contributions in the delivery of patient care. One of those recommendations stressed the importance of academic progression to ensure nurses achieved the highest levels of education available to them to deliver higher levels of quality care and further stipulated that 80% of the nation's nurses should attain a baccalaureate degree by the year 2020 (IOM, 2010).

So, how far have we come over the last 10 years to achieve greater nursing academic progression, specifically the registered nurse to bachelor of science in nursing pathway? The short answer is quite far! There have been multidimensional efforts that led to unprecedented outcomes, namely a 236% increase in RN to BSN graduates from 2009 to 2019 (Campaign for Action, 2021), the development of community college and university partnerships, an overall increase in the number of baccalaureate-prepared nurses from 50% in 2008 to 63% in 2018 (US Department of Health and Human Services, Health Resources and

Services Administration [HRSA], 2018), and the transition of the Robert Wood Johnson Foundation Academic Progression in Nursing to the National Education Progression in Nursing (NEPIN) Collaborative, a movement focused on higher levels of education and achievement for nurses (NEPIN, 2022). These efforts built greater momentum to pursue nursing academic progression.

> *"Creating inclusive learning environments and a more diverse nursing workforce is critical to addressing healthcare disparities and health inequities. All students benefit from exposure to different cultures, perspectives, and experiences during the educational process. Evidence shows that diverse teams outperform homogeneous ones and develop more innovative solutions to complex problems."*
>
> –Deborah Trautman, PhD, RN, FAAN
> President and Chief Executive Officer, American Association of Colleges of Nursing

Unfortunately, that momentum came to a screeching halt in 2020, when the world was shattered by the unprecedented onset of the COVID-19 pandemic. Nurses were suddenly cast onto the worldwide stage as the most trusted pillars of the healthcare system who embodied courage and resiliency during the darkest days of the pandemic. However, COVID-19 took a significant toll on the nursing profession. Not only were lives lost and families destroyed by the pandemic, but the extremely disturbing events that occurred across the country further exacerbated the strain on our collective psyche and exposed the devasting impact that racial and social inequities have on the health and well-being of our nation. The COVID-19 pandemic highlighted the severe toll that structural racism, inherent in our nation's healthcare system, has on health outcomes for individuals of diverse ethnic and racialized backgrounds. Black/AfricanAmerican, Indigenous, and Latinx people disproportionately experienced higher rates of infection, hospitalization, and death when compared with white Americans (Centers for Disease Control and Prevention, 2021; Khazanchi et al., 2021).

The nursing workforce continues to be confronted with a myriad of challenges. However, with adversity comes opportunities that should not be overlooked. It is time community college nursing programs are recognized for the significant role they play in solving the challenges facing our nation's healthcare system. Associate Degree Nursing (ADN) graduates reflect the rich diversity of our communities, representing a wide range of racial, ethnic, gender, sexual orientation, and socioeconomic backgrounds as well as first-generation college graduates. Community college nursing programs provide an essential entry point into the nursing profession, offering an accessible, affordable, high-quality education that lays a solid foundation for future baccalaureate and higher degree obtainment.

As stated in *The Future of Nursing 2020–2030: Charting a Path to Achieve Health Equity*, "health equity is a core component of nursing" (National Academies of Sciences, Engineering, and Medicine [NASEM], 2021, p. 199). Achieving health equity through nursing can be accomplished as "nurses reflect the people and communities served throughout the nation, helping to ensure that individuals receive culturally competent, equitable healthcare services" (NASEM, 2021, p. 3). Most new nursing graduates from diverse backgrounds are entering the nursing profession through community college nursing education programs and the associate degree pathway (Campaign for Action, 2022). In fact, roughly 50% of the entire nursing workforce received their initial nursing education in community colleges and associate degree nursing programs (HRSA, 2018). Community college programs are embedded in local communities and are acutely aware of the residents' unique needs. As a result, graduates of these ADN programs possess a keen understanding of the social determinants of health affecting the population they serve. As critical healthcare providers to marginalized populations, across all care settings, these nurses are prepared to address racial and social inequities and treat the social determinants of health in their professional practices.

The year 2020 was a brutal wake-up call for our nation. The pandemic revealed communities of color were disproportionately impacted by this deadly disease. It exposed the painful truth of how pervasive and deeply embedded structural racism is within our society. Accordingly, community college nursing graduates have proven their ability to be part of the solution in our collective effort to achieve health equity and deliver high-quality care to their communities. As ADN graduates progress to higher levels of education, their communities will continue to reap the benefits of their expertise, knowledge, and abilities.

Prioritizing a highly educated, diverse nursing workforce is imperative for the health and well-being of all Americans. Universities, community colleges, and clinical practice partners must join forces to collectively advance nursing academic progression and ensure associate degree nurses can attain the expanded competencies acquired through baccalaureate education with seamless progression to graduate and doctoral degrees. Recognizing the importance of community college nursing education and advocating for greater inclusivity within all nursing education sends a powerful message that we are working together to achieve our shared goals. Now is the time to collectively move forward and acknowledge that all pathways into the nursing profession are essential to meet the future healthcare needs of all Americans.

References

Campaign for Action. (2021, September 15). *Number of RN-to-BSN program graduates annually.* https://campaignforaction.org/resource/number-rn%E2%80%90to%E2%80%90bsn-graduates-annually/

Campaign for Action. (2022, March 10). *New RN graduates by degree type, by race/ethnicity.* https://campaignforaction.org/resource/new-rn-graduates-degree-type-raceethnicity/

Centers for Disease Control and Prevention. (2021). *Introduction to COVID-19 racial and ethnic health disparities.* https://www.cdc.gov/healthequity/racism-disparities/index.html

Institute of Medicine. (2010). *The future of nursing: Leading change, advancing health.* The National Academies Press. https://doi.org/10.17226/12956

Khazanchi, R., Winkelman, T. N., Pandita, D., Jelinek, R., Shearer, R. D., & Bodurtha, P. J. (2021). Patient characteristics and subsequent health care use by location of SARS-CoV-2 testing initiation in a safety-net health system. *JAMA Network Open, 4*(6), e2112857–e2112857. https://doi.org/10.1001/jamanetworkopen.2021.12857

National Academies of Sciences, Engineering, and Medicine. (2021). *The future of nursing 2020–2030: Charting a path to achieve health equity.* The National Academies Press. https://nam.edu/publications/the-future-of-nursing-2020-2030

National Education Progression in Nursing. (2022). *About.* https://nepincollaborative.org/

US Department of Health and Human Services, Health Resources and Services Administration. (2018). *2018 National Sample Survey of Registered Nurses: Brief summary of results.* https://bhw.hrsa.gov/sites/default/files/bureau-health-workforce/data-research/nssrn-summary-report.pdf

Progressing Beyond Holistic Admissions: Promoting Student Success to Transform the Nursing Workforce

Linda D. Scott, PhD, RN, NEA-BC, FNAP, FAAN
Dean and Professor, University of Wisconsin-Madison School of Nursing

Across the United States, ethnic and racial minorities and other marginalized groups experience significant health disparities as evidenced by lower quality of care, disproportionate healthcare services, and higher mortality rates. Despite an urgent call to diversify health professions made nearly two decades ago by the Institute of Medicine, an adequate response remains unrealized. The absence of a systematic approach to mitigating health disparities reinforces inequities. Moreover, it leaves communities and populations marginalized and with too many unmet needs, requiring us to act on solutions we know can create change.

It has been well documented that having healthcare providers who represent the populations they serve increases access to healthcare and decreases health inequities. This is due to many factors, including that care providers from minoritized groups are more likely to practice in communities of historically excluded individuals (Association of American Medical Colleges, 2014). Additionally, greater improvements in patient outcomes have been demonstrated when patients are treated by providers from similar backgrounds (Cooper et al., 2003; Traylor et al., 2010).

"Excellence in nursing education is a lifelong journey of searching, knowing, implementing, and assessing. Without diversity and inclusion, the search is halfhearted, the knowing has insurmountable walls of unconscious biases, the implementation is restricted by microaggression and structural racism, and the assessment is already prejudiced in its initial design. True excellence in nursing education requires the courage to confront, engage, own, and work with issues of health equity that interfere with the delivery of quality care to all."

–Beverly Malone, PhD, RN, FAAN
Chief Executive Officer, National League for Nursing

Even with an overwhelming need and clear evidence to support the benefits of developing a representative healthcare workforce, meaningful progress is long overdue. Understanding and meeting future workforce needs is a responsibility that motivates academic nurse leaders. While many efforts are in place to advance this, we must continue to expand and evolve our approaches. Our frameworks must promote student success and well-being if we dare set our sights on transformation of—and for— the nursing workforce.

Holistic admission is widely recognized as a strategy to increase diversity in nursing programs and the nursing profession. It relies on more broadly identifying individuals who will make the best nurses. In doing so, holistic admission balances a student's academic metrics with their attributes and experiences. Acknowledging the value of these factors in the context of meeting health needs is a significant and relevant improvement to outdated approaches to student admission processes. Such models isolate and heavily weight academic performance, which—regardless of whether high or low—may be unrelated to a student's aptitude for the nursing profession or their ability to thrive as a student and in their career. In contrast, holistic admission in nursing education factors in the needs and demands of the nursing workforce and the profession overall. This concept has been embraced by nursing programs, and in recent years many schools and colleges have implemented this admission practice.

Positive outcomes in diversity of admission cohorts are typically gained from use of holistic admission processes. While this is essential to achieving a more diverse workforce and improving health for all, the process itself is merely a mechanism to unlock the doors to enrollment. Alone, its benefit to students, nursing programs, and the workforce cannot be fully achieved. Admission and enrollment are simply points along the journey, or life cycle, of a nursing student. Without deliberate approaches to the practices of promoting student success, nursing programs may underserve their students. That is a detriment to *all* students.

Too commonly there is a negative assumption that an outcome of holistic admission is a nursing student population that is "more at risk" for failure. Thus, a second assumption is that remediation support services must be in place for these students. To the contrary, research has found that the overall admission grade point averages are consistently equal or higher among cohorts selected using a holistic admission process compared to those selected without holistic practices in place (Urban Universities for HEALTH, 2014; Zerwic et al., 2018). Nonetheless, negative stereotypes related to diverse and historically excluded students remain unchanged. Through that biased lens, some students seeking assistance may be incorrectly perceived as struggling or at risk when, in fact, they are simply using available resources.

A critical question is whether there is a need to distinguish between what drives one student's need for support, as opposed to what leads another to seek help. I would argue that it does not matter. At least, not if the overall school culture and approach to student services is deliberately and thoughtfully placed on promoting student success. Specifically, this refers to using holistic approaches and factoring in social determinants for success for *all* students.

Nursing education is academically rigorous, emotionally taxing, logistically complicated, and even physically demanding. It is as much a lifestyle as a major, and it can be isolating. Combined, these realities can further exacerbate financial stress and negatively impact physical and emotional well-being for any student. This holds true regardless of whether they are identified or perceived as at-risk at the point of admission, or at any stage of the life cycle in their nursing education. After all, given what we know about the challenges that students face in nursing education, one's designation as struggling (or not) is neither a constant state nor atypical.

To meet the demands of nursing education and the future nursing workforce, there is a need to adjust our attention, approaches, and resources for student success and well-being. Removing the well-intended lens of identifying support systems for at-risk students and replacing it with the culture and practices of promoting student success would benefit all students. Importantly, it would also eliminate harmful assumptions over who does—and who does not—need support.

Transformation is possible if we view the sequence of recruitment, admission, retention, and graduation of students differently than we have in the past. What if we approached the student experience as a holistic process aimed at developing the breadth of nurses needed to meet diverse health needs, while also promoting the health and well-being of themselves and each other? I believe that if we do, then our graduates will be positioned to impact health and thrive in ways that our nursing workforce has yet to achieve.

References

Association of American Medical Colleges. (2014). *Analyzing physician workforce racial and ethnic composition associations: Geographic distribution (part II)*. https://www.aamc.org/media/7621/download

Cooper, L. A., Roter, D. L., Johnson, R. L., Ford, D. E., Steinwachs, D. M., & Powe, N. R. (2003). Patient-centered communication, ratings of care, and concordance of patient and physician race. *Annals of Internal Medicine, 139*(11), 907–915. https://doi.org/10.7326/0003-4819-139-11-200312020-00009

Traylor, A. H., Schmittdiel, J. A., Uratsu, C. S., Mangione, C. M., & Subramanian, U. (2010). Adherence to cardiovascular disease medications: Does patient-provider race/ethnicity and language concordance matter? *Journal of General Internal Medicine, 25*(11), 1172–1177. https://doi.org/10.1007/s11606-010-1424-8

Urban Universities for HEALTH. (2014). *Holistic admissions in the health professions.* https://www.aplu.org/members/commissions/urban-serving-universities/student-success/HolisticAdmissions.pdf

Zerwic, J. J., Scott, L. D., McCreary, L. L., & Corte, C. (2018). Programmatic evaluation of holistic admissions: The influence on students. *Journal of Nursing Education, 57*(7), 416–421. https://doi.org/10.3928/01484834-20180618-06

A Tool to Promote Cultural Humility to Advance Academic Success for American Indian/Alaska Native Nursing Students

Regina Eddie, PhD, MSN, RN
Assistant Professor, Northern Arizona University School of Nursing
Diversity Nursing Consultant, Center to Champion Nursing in America

Nursing is a profession that has long asserted that in order to provide safe, effective and quality care, nurses must first have respect for others, their needs, values, and uniqueness. This assertion is more important than ever given the growing diversity in today's society and requires nursing education to improve the quality of nursing education for diverse nursing students (American Association of Colleges of Nursing [AACN], 2017).

The Campaign for Action's report (2022) tracking new nurse graduates (associate's, bachelor's, and master's programs) by race/ethnicity shows slow progress on increasing the number of nurse graduates across various minoritized groups including Blacks, Asians, and Hispanics but not American Indians/Alaska Natives (AI/ANs). Despite any initiatives, if implemented, by nursing programs to graduate more AI/AN nurses, the number of AI/AN graduates remains stagnant and unchanged. This calls for a deeper look and action to better understand and create a learning environment that is needed to support, retain, and graduate more AI/AN nurse graduates to improve the underrepresentation of AI/AN nurses in our nation's largest healthcare profession.

As an enrolled member of the Diné (Navajo) Nation and one of few AI, PhD-trained nurse educators, I find myself in a unique position to be a voice and advocate for AI nursing students. I begin by asking the following questions: Why have we not been able to see better results in graduation rates for AI/AN students? What type of education pathways can make it easier for students to be successful? And lastly, how can we admit more AI/AN students into nursing programs?

At the root of what is needed is a learning environment that embraces and improves a better understanding of AI students, their cultural background, and the influence of culture on life and learning experiences, attitudes, and beliefs. This is important to highlight given the body of evidence that suggests diverse students, including AI students, often face many difficulties in a learning environment, challenging their path to academic success, progression, and successful completion. Such challenges well documented in the literature include financial hardships, a disconnect with peers and faculty (which is compounded by lack of cultural understanding and sensitivity), difficulties with transitioning to the academic setting due to feelings of isolation, an unwelcoming environment, prejudice, and racism (Cech et al., 2011).

To move toward a more inclusive learning environment, a focus on cultural humility is gaining more attention and acceptance in nursing education as an integral strategy for valuing and respecting diverse nursing students. Yet, many nursing faculty struggle with how to promote or practice it (Smith & Foronda, 2021). *Cultural humility* is defined as having traits of respect, empathy, an openness to learn about other perspectives and cultures, and to engage in self-reflection (Foronda et al., 2016) to differences in sexual preference, social status, interprofessional roles, to healthcare provider/patient relationships. The attributes were openness, self-awareness, egolessness, supportive interactions, and self-reflection and critique. The antecedents were diversity and power imbalance. The consequences were mutual empowerment, partnerships, respect, optimal care, and lifelong learning. Cultural humility was described as a lifelong process. With a firm understanding of the term, individuals and communities will be better equipped to understand and accomplish an inclusive environment with mutual benefit and optimal care (Foronda et al., 2016). Applying cultural humility can help nurse educators build trusting relationships and help students feel supported in their learning experience. Mentoring, particularly one that is culturally tailored, is one approach to foster a strong relationship with AI/AN students. Mentoring has long been deemed an important strategy to support academic success.

In 2020, the *Future of Nursing: Campaign for Action*, an initiative by the AARP Foundation, AARP, the Robert Wood Johnson Foundation, and the National Alaska Native American Indian Nurses Association (NANAINA) launched an important and collaborative undertaking to help create a more holistic, supportive, and caring learning environment for AI/AN nursing students through a mentoring curriculum resource that was developed for nursing faculty. This effort continues as part of ongoing work to help address the underrepresentation of AI/AN nurses and improve health equity in AI communities. The collaborative effort, sponsored by Campaign for Action, brought together various Native American (and non-Native) nurse leaders from schools of nursing education programs, NANAINA, Indian Health Services, and the AACN for their expertise to develop and implement a first-of-its-kind mentoring curriculum to support culturally tailored mentoring of AI/AN nursing students.

The curriculum, titled "Pathways to Promote Academic Success for American Indian/Alaska Native Nursing Students: A Mentoring Curriculum for Nursing Faculty," was completed in May 2021 (Campaign for Action, 2021b). The mentoring curriculum is designed to help nursing faculty understand the unique needs of AI/AN nursing students and be better prepared to support and promote academic success, retention, and graduation of students. The objectives of the AI/AN mentoring curriculum include the following:

- Provide an overview of AI/AN historical, social, and political context and its influence on higher education experiences

- Impart guidance on culturally sensitive and responsive mentoring approaches and teaching/learning strategies for faculty

- Provide guidance on strategies to support AI/AN student retention and academic success

- Present information and resources on approaches for recruitment of AI/AN students

The curriculum has five main sections that begin with an overview of AI/AN historical, social, and political context, and contain a comprehensive mentoring plan that is divided into seven culturally relevant categories and includes specific teaching/learning strategies for how faculty can support academic success for AI/AN students. Additionally, the curriculum resource offers recruitment strategies for schools of nursing to consider, including holistic admissions.

This new culturally tailored tool was introduced as part of Campaign for Action's ongoing work to increase diversity in the nursing workforce by supporting mentoring training to nursing programs. The mentor training, "Diversifying the Nursing Workforce: Mentoring for Student Retention and NCLEX Success at American Indian/Alaska Native–Serving Institutions," was held virtually in September 2021 (Campaign for Action, 2021a). Thirty Native American–serving school of nursing programs were represented at the training. The recording of the two-day virtual webinar along with the AI/AN mentoring curriculum is available publicly on the Campaign for Action website and can be used to improve the learning experience for AI/AN nursing students.

References

American Association of Colleges of Nursing. (2017). *Diversity, equity, and inclusion in academic nursing*. https://www.aacnnursing.org/News-Information/Position-Statements-White-Papers/Diversity

Campaign for Action. (2021a). *Diversifying the nursing workforce: Mentoring for student retention and NCLEX success at American Indian/Alaska Native-serving institutions*. https://campaignforaction.org/webinar/mentoring-at-ai-an-serving-institutions/

Campaign for Action. (2021b). *Pathways to promote academic success for American Indian/Alaska Native nursing students: A mentoring curriculum for nursing faculty*. https://campaignforaction.org/resource/ai-an-mentoring-curriculum-for-nursing-faculty/

Campaign for Action. (2022). *New RN graduates by degree type, by race/ethnicity*. https://campaignforaction.org/resource/new-rn-graduates-degree-type-raceethnicity/

Cech, E. A., Metz, A. M., Babcock, T., & Smith, J. L. (2011). Caring for our own: The role of institutionalized support structures in Native American nursing student success. *Journal of Nursing Education, 50*(9), 524–531. https://doi.org/10.3928/01484834-20110517-01

Foronda, C., Baptiste, D.-L., Reinholdt, M. M., & Ousman, K. (2016). Cultural humility: A concept analysis. *Journal of Transcultural Nursing, 27*(3), 210–217. https://doi.org/10.1177/1043659615592677

Smith, A., & Foronda, C. (2021). Promoting cultural humility in nursing education through the use of ground rules. *Nursing Education Perspectives, 42*(2), 117–119. https://doi.org/10.1097/01.NEP.0000000000000594

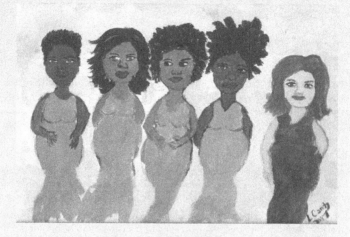

The Invitation

I was invited to the party
But I was not allowed to dance
While the movements were beautiful
I realized I could not see any traces of myself
Where was I in this sequence of expressions
How could I fit in when I never learned the steps?
As the dance became more complex
I could see myself floating further and further away

I was given a seat at the table
But I wasn't allowed to speak
Expected to sit quietly while others spoke their truth
Using a language that I never understood
Words so eloquent I could not see them
eradicating my existence.

My silence signified an acceptance I never consented to
My contributions made absent in this never-ending story.
My challenges never heard
My story never told
It is as though I do not exist
Maybe, just maybe
I was not expected to accept the invitation

Poetry and artwork by Lucinda Canty, PhD, CNM, FACNM
Associate Professor of Nursing, University of Massachusetts Amherst

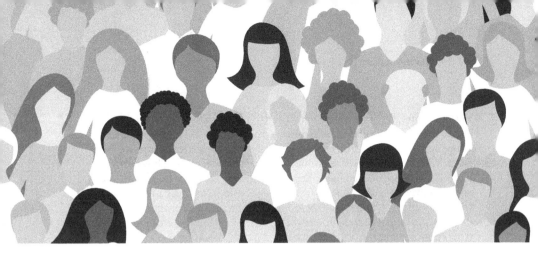

3 Diversity and Mentorship

In This Chapter

In this chapter, the importance of diversifying the nursing workforce and leadership in academic and clinical settings is examined, as well as the significance of mentorship. Overall, the nursing profession has consistently improved upon diversifying the workforce regarding direct patient/client care; however, that goal has been far more challenging when considering diversity in leadership. Sharing and acknowledging the perspectives and experiences of nurses and student nurses who face barriers to advancement in their careers provides insight on how to diversify nursing. Additionally, providing dependable, intentional mentorship can offer opportunities for exposure, sponsorship, and coaching to create a sustainable pipeline to achieve diversity at every career level and specialty in the nursing profession.

Consider the following questions as you read the essays about health equity and diversity and mentorship:

- What are important systemic or institutional changes that can be implemented to increase diversity?

- What are steps in an effective strategy to diversify the nursing profession and improve health equity?

- What are ways for a mentor to support a mentee?

- How can nurses work to improve diversity in academic and clinical settings?

- In what ways can nursing programs provide meaningful support to people from minoritized and disadvantaged backgrounds?

Students Who Look Like Me

Wallena "Lena" Gould, EdD, CRNA, FAANA, FAAN
Founder & Chief Executive Officer, Diversity in Nurse Anesthesia Mentorship Program

Professional socialization for early career nurses is critical (van Rooyen et al., 2018). However, nurses who have been historically marginalized may not experience the same inclusion and belonging needed to achieve career advancement (Iheduru-Anderson, 2020). This declarative statement was almost not delivered due to racial bias, redlining, inequities in educational opportunities, and racism embedded in nursing programs.

Over 35 years ago, after graduating high school in New Jersey as a young Black single teenage mother, I was suddenly homeless with no telephone or computer access. Economic instability and social environment are some of the social determinants that adversely impacted my educational and professional growth (Sanderson et al., 2021). Structural determinants and institutional barriers negatively impacted my transition into nursing and my professional advancement as a nurse anesthetist. We were homeless for three months, and the public library became a place of refuge while I made daily visits to the housing authority hoping for a rent-subsidized apartment. Finally, I secured a one-bedroom apartment with $273 of state cash assistance, $114 worth of food stamps, and Medicaid.

In undergraduate school, I was interested in nursing, but I could not pass the SAT exam, and I did not have reliable transportation for clinical. These structural barriers and other financial constraints created significant challenges for completing a degree in nursing. In addition to limited resources, first-generation college students also struggle with how to navigate academic settings because of a lack of generational knowledge. Nursing school was not encouraged in my urban high school, and admission into a rigorous program of study seemed unattainable. Traditionally open doors of opportunity were often closed for students like me.

Despite many barriers, I graduated with high academic honors with a degree in accounting. After working one year as an auditor, I decided this was not the right career for me. I changed my professional trajectory and decided to explore a future in nursing. I decided to apply to an associate degree in nursing program because of accessibility. Again, I excelled academically and passed the boards on the first attempt. My first nursing position was in the operating room, where I had the opportunity to work with nurse anesthetists. In nursing school, I was not encouraged to further my education and become an advanced practice nurse, nor did I have any nursing faculty who looked like me to serve as role models. Notably, I worked with a Black woman, a chief CRNA, who was a role model for me.

A few years later, I left the operating room to gain requisite skills needed in telemetry and trauma unit so I could apply to a nurse anesthesia program. My acceptance in the nurse anesthesia program should have been celebratory, but I was only granted conditional acceptance due to my GRE score. In my admission letter, I was told that I had to register for six credits of graduate nursing courses and earn at least a B grade to receive full acceptance. For the next year, I worked full time while taking 15 credits of graduate level pre-requisite courses and earned an exemplary grade in each class before matriculating into the nurse anesthesia program. My GRE score was not a valid indicator of my academic ability or potential for success in the CRNA program.

As a matriculated nurse anesthesia student in Philadelphia, I noticed the nurse anesthesia faculty and student cohorts did not resemble the community we served. During my studies, a poster project was assigned, and I choose to focus on "Diversity in Nurse Anesthesia." Marian Wright Edelman, founder of the Children's Defense Fund, coined the phrase, "You can't be what you can't see." I took this to heart and made sure images of nurse anesthesia students of color were prominently placed in the poster.

I graduated from the nurse anesthesia program with high academic honors and passed the CRNA boards on my first attempt. While many nurses of color experience a lack of belonging and mentorship, I was provided mentorship from two strong nurse anesthesia leaders, Goldie Brangman and Dr. Arthur Zwerling. Both nursing luminaries helped light a path for me and contributed significantly to my socialization as a CRNA. They inspired me to be a mentor, too. That poster project on diversity eventually turned into a nonprofit organization and is now an exemplar initiative, Immersion Model for Diversifying the Nurse Anesthesia Programs (Gould, 2021). This model program has led to over 658 nurses of color entering and graduating from 92 nurse anesthesia programs. Today, they are CRNAs, PhD researchers, and Fellows of the American Academy of Nursing. They light the path for other diverse nurses to become CRNAs.

To remove barriers and increase the number of diverse nurse anesthetists, I recommend the following actions:

1. Eliminate SATs and GREs as admission criteria into nursing programs and adopt a holistic admission policy.

2. Recruit and retain nursing and nurse anesthesia faculty and clinical coordinators of color.

3. Develop bridge programs for associate degree in nursing graduates for direct entry into DNP or DNAP nurse anesthesia programs to reduce unnecessary financial debt.

4. Invite diverse CRNA professionals to be paid guest lecturers or serve as adjunct professors.

5. Develop an anti-racist curriculum in nursing schools, and employ diverse nurses to teach such content.

6. Create pipeline mentorship programs with emphasis on early professional socialization.

7. Increase the number of systematically marginalized, PhD-prepared nurse researchers with HRSA and NIH grants awarded to nurses of color.

8. Collect data on microaggressions, encountered racism, and attrition rates of students of color, with public reporting systems for accountability.

9. Intentionally partner with Historically Black Colleges and Universities, Hispanic-Serving Institutions, and American Indian/Alaskan Native schools of nursing with shared resources and active mentoring of students and faculty.

As a Black woman in a predominantly white profession, I want to echo the remarks by Senator Cory Booker to Judge Ketanji Brown Jackson at her Supreme Court confirmation hearing: "Don't worry, my sister, God has got you. I know what it took for you to get here."

References

Gould, W. (2021). Historical underpinning to diversifying nurse anesthesia programs: A model of success. *Teaching and Learning in Nursing, 16*(2), 175–180. https://doi.org/10.1016/j.teln.2020.11.004

Iheduru-Anderson, K. (2020). Barriers to career advancement in the nursing profession: Perceptions of Black nurses in the United States. *Nursing Forum, 55*(4), 664–677. https://doi.org/10.1111/nuf.12483

Sanderson, C. D., Hollinger-Smith, L. M., & Cox, K. (2021). Developing a Social Determinants of Learning™ framework: A case study. *Nursing Education Perspectives, 42*(4), 205–211. https://doi.org/10.1097/01.NEP.0000000000000810

van Rooyen, D. R., Jordan, P. J., ten Ham-Baloyi, W., & Caka, E. M. (2018). A comprehensive literature review of guidelines facilitating transition of newly graduated nurses to professional nurses. *Nurse Education in Practice, 30*, 35–41. https://doi.org/10.1016/j.nepr.2018.02.010

Diversity in Mentorship and Sponsorship for Nursing Leadership Development

Jing Wang, PhD, MPH, RN, FAAN
Dean and Professor, Florida State University College of Nursing

Diversity in mentorship and sponsorship has played an essential role in my career growth and development as a nurse leader. Such diversity spans over age, gender, race, ethnicity, professional affiliations, senior/peer mentors, culture, urban/rural region, and many more. When I was a BSN-PhD student at the University of Pittsburgh School of Nursing, Dr. Villarruel, then the President of the National Coalition of Ethnic Minority Nurses Association (NCEMNA), emailed me and asked me to speak at a convention when I was selected as an NCEMNA Mentee. It was the first time that I learned about mentorship, and I received advice from mentors at NCEMNA to go beyond just my own ethnic and racial groups and study the most underserved populations. I have since then embarked on my own nursing research career studying technology among the most historically excluded and frail populations from underserved areas. Fifteen years later, I am proud to serve on the board of directors at NCEMNA and as President of the Asian American/Pacific Islander Nurses Association (AAPINA), working closely with leaders from other ethnic minority organizations including the National Alaska Native American Indian Nurses Association (NANAINA), the National Association of Hispanic Nurses (NAHN), the National Black Nurses Association (NBNA), and the Philippine Nurses Association of America (PNAA). I am inspired every day by these minoritized nurse leaders who have been volunteering to serve the profession and their communities with countless hours of their personal time to advocate for health equity. I had the privilege to be mentored by many but want to call out two late minoritized leaders whose legacy I am pleased to see continued at the national level devoted to mentorship: Yu (Philip) Xu Mentoring Award at AAPINA, and Duck-Hee Kang Memorial Mentored Workshop for Early Career Nurse Scientists at the Council for the Advancement of Nursing Science (CANS).

Standing on the shoulders of many giant leaders and becoming the Dean at Florida State University (FSU) College of Nursing, I have the great opportunity to embark on new initiatives to diversify a nursing pipeline at an academic institution through problem-solving of the root causes of lack of diversity in our nursing student applicant pools. We quickly expanded our outreach program through partnership with the FSU College of Medicine's Science Students Together Reaching Instructional Diversity & Excellence (SSTRIDE) program. STRIDE operates as a pipeline program and provides resources to students from traditionally underserved and historically excluded backgrounds in middle schools and high schools across the state of Florida. The program provides in-school and afterschool support services; however, the program has not traditionally incorporated a nursing component. Through a grant from our Office of Diversity and Inclusion, we were able to host several nursing workshops and tours to engage SSTRIDE students. Additionally, we worked with our local Boys and Girls Club to host workshops and afterschool tours with assistance from the Center for Academic Retention and Enhancement (CARE) program, which provides academic support and programming for first generation and underserved populations at both pre-collegiate and collegiate levels. We hope to continue fostering relationships and allocating resources to help expand our reach to communities that have not traditionally been a part of our applicant pool, as well as peer mentoring to support their successes in their pre-nursing and pre-college years. These efforts will aid us in identifying high-achieving, unrecognized students for whom we are able to provide tuition support through our newly established innovative academic practice initiatives for those in need.

"The lack of nurse leaders from diverse backgrounds is a major obstacle to fully realizing our profession's commitment to advancing health equity. Mentorship is a key component of efforts to attract and retain a diverse nursing workforce. There is a need for targeted mentorship programs to ensure that individuals from minoritized backgrounds receive the resources and support they need to succeed in nursing."

–Billy Caceras, PhD, RN, FAHA, FAAN
Assistant Professor, School of Nursing at Columbia University

Diversity in mentoring of historically excluded and diverse faculty in academic institutions is also critical to ensure that students from diverse backgrounds have opportunities to work with role models from similar backgrounds. Through one of the first six awards and only one led by a college of nursing, funded by the first round of the National Institute of Health Common Fund's Faculty Institutional Recruitment for Sustainable Transformation (FIRST) program, aiming to "enhance and maintain cultures of inclusive excellence in the biomedical research community" (NIH Common Fund, 2022, para. 1). I had the opportunity as a Dean to support our research center directors with decades of experience supporting "inclusive excellence" to establish cultures that develop and sustain scientific environments that will cultivate and benefit from a full range of talent. The training and mentoring I received from diverse leaders had prepared me to advocate for a diverse nursing research pipeline working on the National Institute of Nursing Research (NINR) Council Working Group on Diversity.

Carefully thought out and planned mentoring, coaching, and leadership development programs are proven to be successful in nursing and healthcare. Throughout my nursing career, I had the opportunity to participate in the Robert Wood Johnson Foundation Nurse Faculty Scholars program, the Josiah Macy Jr. Foundation Macy Faculty Scholars program, and the Health and Aging Policy Fellows program. All these programs have very structured mentoring and were developed by thoughtful leaders committed to diversity. I would not be bold enough to take on any leadership roles I am currently holding without these life-changing programs. I feel so comfortable now making risky yet needed decisions, working with other professions, working through conflicts, and sometimes putting myself in uncomfortable situations. So many nursing and healthcare leaders have mentored and supported me in my career; they empower me to lead, give back, and mentor the next generation of nurses and nurse leaders. Being mentored and encouraged to take on leadership roles at local, national, and global levels, I am often reminded by the mentors and sponsors from diverse backgrounds that contributed to my learning and growth. I am forever grateful to the many great mentors. They have shown me the power of diverse people working together to achieve excellence in health and healthcare through diversity, for our beloved nursing profession and for the patients and communities we serve and love dearly to have fair and just opportunities to a culture of health and quality healthcare.

Reference

NIH Common Fund. (2022). *Faculty Institutional Recruitment for Sustainable Transformation (FIRST)*. National Institutes of Health. https://commonfund.nih.gov/first

Mentoring to Diversify

Derrick T. McCoy, Jr., BSN, RN
Registered Nurse, Grady Health

I began my nursing career in 2020 as a nurse extern in a small rural hospital with just 14 ICU beds. At the time, I was one of two staff members of color providing care to a population that did not look like me. Suddenly, the only person I could relate to vanished without any notice, leaving me in panic. All eyes were on me. If I sat too long, I was lazy. If I disagreed with a doctor, I was labeled insubordinate. Literally and figuratively, I was the black sheep.

> *"Diversity mentoring helps an organization identify the similarities within a diverse workforce and leverage them to build a united workforce with common goals. Diversity mentoring also helps to further unite the workforce by recognizing differences as an opportunity to learn and grow. Mentoring results in learning and growing together, sharing experiences and knowledge. It is a highly effective method to support diversity and inclusion in an organization. Mentorship unlocks the power of diversity and inclusion."*
>
> —Reynaldo R. Rivera, DNP, RN, NEA-BC, FAAN
> Director of Nursing Research and Innovation, New York-Presbyterian Hospital
> Assistant Professor of Clinical Nursing, Columbia University School of Nursing

Then the COVID-19 pandemic struck, and this once 14-bed ICU was now home to 24 ICU beds. Along with this addition came an increase of travel nurses from across the United States, providing not only relief for the hospital but for me as well. I no longer found myself looking over my shoulder as the constant arrival of more nurses of color entered this unit providing the best care available. Almost immediately, I became exposed to more of what the world and the nursing profession had to offer.

The leaders I met and mentors I gained were essential to who I am now. Diversity and mentoring in the nursing profession plays a pivotal role in any nurse's success; however, the future of nursing is uncertain, as we are far from meeting our diversity standard and increasing mentorship.

Every hospital has a short section in their onboarding presentation titled "Diversity and Inclusion." The PowerPoint slide will have a photo of three individuals in scrubs, all from different ethnic backgrounds, and all smiling with their perfect white teeth. The onboarding personnel will then present a Google images search result for "diversity in healthcare" and will say, "Diversity matters." However, when the new employees get a tour of the unit, they see the real-world "diversity"—nothing that compares to the photos shown in the presentation. It is a false reassurance that even novice nursing students are told to avoid because it is something not based on fact. Instead of making fictitious claims about how diversity matters, the statement should read "Representation matters." A strong and positive representation helps by deteriorating the stereotypes that may hinder a minoritized society. Representation begets diversity.

So, is there one solution or some overarching plan to increase diversity in healthcare? I do not think so; however, one thing that has guided me through a flawed diversity system is mentorship. As I began my collegiate career in nursing, I met my first mentor, Dr. LaDonia Patterson. Her creativity, inspiration, and strategic vision were just a few of the traits she possessed—she was a beacon of representation that supported a dream I could not imagine for myself. Furthermore, a mentor from an ethnic minority who engages with you and establishes a mentor-mentee relationship provides formal access to executive leadership and opportunities that may not have been easily attainable. This relationship provides connections to positions of leadership and allows the members at the highest level of command to become more diverse. With diverse leadership, the culture of the hospital changes. The level of diversity that can be seen at the highest level of the hospital, such as the Director of Nursing, CEO, and CFO, changes the image of the hospital, allowing the hospital community to target each minoritized group.

Thankfully, mentorship has molded my career and provided me with the skill set and confidence to face obstacles head-on, even when diversity is not abundant, instead of giving up and changing paths. I have taken those obstacles and used the lessons learned from them to navigate toward my goal. Dr. Patterson's knowledge and experience opened my eyes to other viewpoints and professional methodologies while still allowing me to stay true to my beliefs. A mentor will allow the mentee to be vulnerable and expressive and provide insight into their own mistakes and mishaps in hopes of saving the mentee time, money, and running the risk of receiving misinformation.

In an industry lacking representation for people of color, it takes a strong-minded, positive, and patient individual to guide the future minds of an industry that will forever be in demand. Achieving diversity in this field will bring growth for the organization by means of personnel or differing ideologies and will also allow for groups of people who have been historically excluded to have a chance to be seen and heard in the same forum and with the same level of respect as their counterparts not represented. Furthermore, this creates a chance to change the healthcare industry as a whole.

How do we continue the daily business of nursing while simultaneously working to strategically and consistently improve diversity in the field? We start by supporting mentors in every healthcare sector, from academia to frontline workers. We allow our mentors to bestow knowledge to those eager to learn and make a difference in a world where a minoritized society constantly struggles to gain acceptance and growth. We encourage authentic representation not from one minoritized group but instead from multiple ethnicities to truly live by those onboarding words, "diversity and inclusion."

One Strategy to Increase Nursing Workforce Diversity

Vernell P. DeWitty, PhD, MBA, RN
Chief Diversity, Equity, and Inclusion Officer, American Association of
Colleges of Nursing

It is generally accepted that the term *mentor* comes from Homer's *Odyssey*, when King Odysseus entrusts the care of his household to a man named Mentor, who serves as teacher and overseer of the royal prince. Today, mentoring is defined as a learning partnership, where the mentor and mentee work collaboratively toward the achievement of mutually defined goals, typically focused on developing a mentee's skills, abilities, and knowledge. In essence, a more experienced or knowledgeable person helps to guide a less experienced or knowledgeable person (Crisp et al., 2017).

Today, mentoring is a buzzword, and the benefits are widely extolled. Mentoring programs in organizations take on many different forms and a variety of purposes. For some organizations, mentoring becomes a strategy for succession planning or talent development and often provides opportunities for recruitment and retention of emerging leaders. Individuals may seek out mentors whom they determine will best help them achieve their career goals and establish long-term learning relationships. Mentors can serve a valuable role in helping guide the development and advancement of nursing students and nurses throughout their career. Most experienced nurses, regardless of professional role, will readily express gratitude and identify the benefits they received through mentoring relationships.

Diversity in the nursing workforce can only be accomplished when more diverse students enroll, advance, and graduate from nursing schools. According to data from the American Association of Colleges of Nursing (AACN, 2022), the percentage of graduates from diverse backgrounds increased by 10% from 2012 to 2022 (26.7% to 36.7%), which is progress. Mentoring is one strategy that supports the success of historically minoritized students and is frequently identified as an essential component to meeting academic goals. There are several key components for establishing a successful mentoring relationship (Ovink & Veazey, 2010):

1. Mentoring is most successful when the partners recognize the strengths and cultural norms associated with students and the focus expands beyond merely the assimilation of students into academic environments.

2. Successful mentoring program implementation requires clarity in purpose and alignment with the organizational culture.

3. The mentor and mentee must establish, early in the relationship, a shared understanding of their assumptions, expectations, and goals. The partners should discuss and agree on ensuring confidentiality, boundaries, and limits.

4. When challenges develop in mentoring relationships, the underlying reasons often stem from the fact that the relationship did not begin with having these important conversations.

The benefits of mentoring should be clearly articulated to mentors and mentees as part of the program design. An introduction and orientation session to mentoring should be offered to promote program success. Frequently, nursing schools identify the lack of mentors as a primary reason for not initiating or sustaining a mentoring program. However, schools may consider recruiting mentors from the community or alumni from the nursing school. It is customary to focus on 1:1 mentoring; however, there are other approaches that are also very effective, such as peer mentoring or group mentoring models. A mentoring toolkit was designed by the New Careers in Nursing Scholarship program to bring a mutual understanding to the process, design, and implementation of mentoring programs. This resource can be customized for a variety of mentoring programs (Robert Wood Johnson Foundation & American Association of Colleges of Nursing, 2016).

The recruitment and retention of diverse faculty remain significant concerns in academia and specifically in nursing. In 2021, the AACN reported a national faculty vacancy rate of 8%, which represents a sharp increase over the 6.5% reported in 2020. The majority of schools reporting vacancies (84.4%) indicated a preference for faculty with doctoral degrees (AACN, 2022). The impact of having too few faculty is significant. Students indicate an enhanced sense of belonging and the desire to see faculty members who look like them.

Most nursing schools recognize the value of increasing the diversity of faculty; however, limited attention is given to removing the barriers identified by earlier research studies (Zambrana et al., 2015). The barriers that contribute to attrition from doctoral programs of study include financial assistance, faculty mentoring, family support, and peer support. Mentoring is one strategy to assist in advancing academic careers and helps racially/ethnically diverse faculty achieve career success by addressing the identity, self-efficacy, and cultural capital that they must develop to navigate research communities of practice.

To strengthen the capacity of the nursing workforce to provide quality care in all communities, nursing schools must educate a more diverse population of students who are prepared to care for an increasingly diverse population. A critical component of the academic advancement and success of a diverse student population is a more diverse nursing school faculty. Academic nursing must attend to both needs simultaneously if we are intentional about increasing health equity for all.

References

American Association of Colleges of Nursing. (2022). *2021–2022 enrollment and graduations in baccalaureate and graduate programs in nursing.* https://www.aacnnursing.org/Store/product-info/productcd/IDSR_22ENROLLBACC

Crisp, G., Baker, V. L., Griffin, K. A., Lunsford, L. G., & Pifer, M. J. (2017). Mentoring undergraduate students. *ASHE Higher Education Report, 43*(1). 7–103. https://doi.org/10.1002/aehe.20117

Ovink, S. M., & Veazey, B. D. (2010) More than "getting us through": A case study in cultural capital enrichment of underrepresented minority undergraduates. *Research in Higher Education, 52,* 370–394.

Robert Wood Johnson Foundation & American Association of Colleges of Nursing. (2016). *The mentoring toolkit and handbook.* Robert Wood Johnson Foundation New Careers in Nursing. http://www.newcareersinnursing.org/resources/mentoring-toolkit-and-handbook.html

Zambrana, R. E., Ray, R., Espino, M. M., Castro, C., Cohen, B. D., & Eliason, J. (2015) "Don't leave us behind": The importance of mentoring underrepresented minority faculty. *American Educational Research Journal, 52*(1), 40–72. https://doi.org/10.3102/0002831214563063

Academia and Practice: Partnering for Diversity

Kathleen Sanford, DBA, RN, FACHE, FAAN
Executive Vice President and Chief Nursing Officer, CommonSpirit Health

I read the book *Difficult Conversations: How to Discuss What Matters Most* when it was first published in 1999. The authors posited that politics, religion, gender, and race may be among the most difficult subjects for people to discuss (Stone et al., 1999). I'm not sure if what followed was a direct result of that book or if the book's timing matched an evolving consciousness among healthcare executives. Whatever the cause, it seemed that, almost overnight, the professional conferences and meetings I attended uniformly started offering breakout sessions on the need to engage in conversations about race and the lack of diversity among healthcare professionals, and particularly, among our healthcare leaders. I remember some specifics from a few of those discussions, just as I recall how uncomfortable some communications were.

It is now 23 years later, and nurse leaders, among others, are still talking. What changes have occurred since we first openly recognized the imbalance between the number of minoritized caregivers, healthcare executives, and the individuals and communities we care for? From my point of view, it appears our conversations today aren't as stilted as they were in those earlier years. There are more voiced acknowledgments that racism and cultural biases are root causes for current societal inequities. Many of our hospitals and systems list both diversity of staff and care equity as important goals for their organizations. Conference speakers and authors correlate quality and patient experience with a diverse staff caring for similarly diverse populations. We seem to "get it" that provider diversity and equity of care are inexorably linked. Yet, our progress in both seems to be slow, considering all that talk, and our human resources partners tell us that they have difficulty recruiting diverse candidates, especially for leadership positions.

A simplified version of an effective strategy to diversify our profession and eliminate inequities in care has three major steps: 1. clear articulation of a vision for the future, 2. an understanding of the current state and how it differs from the vision, and 3. implementation of specific tactics to bridge the gap between the vision and current state. The statistics shared above describe our current state. From my perspective, we have completed steps 1 and 2, and step 3 is where nurse leaders should be concentrating our efforts today. We need to then share the results of our tactics with each other so we can learn which are best practices on our strategic journey to diversification and health equity. We also need to find and collaborate with partners who share our vision.

An Example of Partnering to Achieve Diversity

Colleges of nursing have long partnered with healthcare organizations for the education and professional development of both undergraduate and graduate nurses. This partnership allows for envisioning and pursuing a future where our efforts can create a more supportive career continuum for nurses from pre-nursing school to wherever an individual's aspirations take them, including executive leadership.

A university and healthcare system could partner to offer that career continuum with a variety of tactics:

- Educating minoritized children and teens on the intrinsic and extrinsic rewards of a nursing career

- Partnering on creative ways to fund nursing education for individual students, including part-time jobs in hospitals with tuition loan forgiveness programs

- Providing mentors and tutors for nursing students from underprivileged backgrounds

- Providing (when possible) clinical nurse preceptors of the same race or ethnicity to work with nursing students during their clinical placement in the healthcare organization

- Increasing the number of college educators through innovative employment and education plans

- Placing newly graduated nurses in clinical residency programs

- Providing tuition reimbursement for pursuance of graduate degrees

- Assigning mentors and/or career counselors

- Including minoritized nurse candidates in succession planning and assigning them growth and education opportunities in preparation to compete for promotions

There are undoubtedly other tactics, but these are on the list to be considered as part of the nascent strategy for the collaboration between CommonSpirit Health and Charles R. Drew University of Medicine and Science. These two entities—a healthcare system striving to improve health while advancing social justice and an institution of higher learning committed to cultivating diverse health professional leaders who are dedicated to social justice and health equity—share three goals. These are:

- To increase the number of nursing graduates in California and assist in the placement of these graduates in areas with identified need

- To increase the diversity of individuals entering and graduating from nursing programs

- To increase the access to education by diverse populations by addressing barriers to educational success and providing access to care in areas that may lack access to healthcare providers.

As we proceed with our strategy to meet those goals, we will share our journey with our nurse colleagues, including the challenges and successes of specific tactics.

Taking Action Now

We still have many difficult conversations ahead of us about the root causes of health inequities in this country. These discussions will continue to be important and will help us gain greater insight into each other, our own biases, how to be more inclusive, and what we can do to change or mitigate current realities caused by past injustice. We have an industry-wide need to increase the cultural competence of all nurses, and we have an ethical and moral imperative to protect our staff from unfair acts (including hurtful communications). Conversations with our team members may help us understand these issues in our own organizations

What we can't do is limit our responsibilities as nurse leaders to conversations. Identified issues need to be addressed. It is time for academia and practice to partner in implementations of concrete strategies and tactics to increase the diversity of nursing as a whole and match the diversity of our nurses and nurse leaders to the diversity of our patients and consumers. To quote multiple sources, "If not us, who? If not now, when?" It will only be nurses who take action to diversify nursing, and we should do it together.

Reference

Stone, D., Patton, B., Heen, S., & Fisher, R. (1999). *Difficult conversations*. Viking.

Mentoring Minoritized Nursing Students in an Anti-Racist Era

Rosa M. Gonzalez-Guarda, PhD, MPH, RN, FAAN
Assistant Dean, PhD Program
Associate Professor, Duke University School of Nursing

The COVID-19 pandemic has amplified deeply rooted inequities in the US to create a new context in which nursing students are prepared to address the most pressing societal problems. In fact, the COVID-19 pandemic increased the demand of healthcare providers to not only be prepared to serve during a state of emergency, but also respond to the inequities that were manifested in the over inclusion of minoritized racial and ethnic groups in COVID-19 infections, hospitalizations, and deaths (Mackey et al., 2021). These inequities in health were co-occurring alongside syndemic social traumas such as the targeted acts of police brutality against Black Americans, the separation of children from their parents at the US-Mexico border, and the increased anti-Asian sentiment that led to an increase in crimes against this population (Elias et al., 2021; Mendenhall et al., 2022; Wilson & Stimpson, 2020). While the toll of the COVID-19 pandemic and the awakening of systemic racism were felt by all nursing students who had to adapt to the changing education and healthcare systems and engage in self-reflection around one's own contribution to and experience with systemic racism, minoritized nursing students were likely disproportionately affected as they experienced a higher burden of loss and suffering based on social conditions associated with their identities.

Strong mentorship of minoritized students, especially by faculty with shared similar racial/ethnic identities, is a well-documented facilitator of success in nursing education (Osakwe et al., 2022). Yet, mentoring within the context of an anti-racist era has not been well defined. Anti-racist frameworks call for policies and actions that directly call out and address overt or covert manifestations of racism. These include (Bell, 2021; Cary et al., 2020; Coleman, 2020):

- Adopting a position that is explicitly anti-racist
- Including everyone as agents of change, not just minoritized faculty, staff, and students who have historically taken the lead on this work

- Ongoing coursework and training for faculty, staff, and students on topics such as health equity; diversity, equity, and inclusion; multiculturalism; power and privilege; intersectionality; and anti-racist bystander behavior

- Fostering community-academic partnerships, especially with historically marginalized communities

- Leveraging transdisciplinary resources from not only health but also the social and political sciences

When integrated with the science of effective mentoring strategies that foster professional and personal support and growth (National Academies of Sciences, Engineering, and Medicine, 2020), the anti-racist context poses unique challenges for mentor-mentee pairs from minoritized groups in nursing.

The increased demand for anti-racist behaviors has supported minoritized students and their mentors to call out mistreatments and injustices they experience. This places minoritized students in a position of vulnerability, where calling out these mistreatments may label them as "difficult" and taint their reputation among both faculty and peers. Mentors providing support to their mentees during these situations may face similar repercussions, especially if they themselves have also been mistreated in that organization and are early career (e.g., non-tenured). Additionally, mentors may also have a low sense of efficacy in engaging in anti-racist behaviors, as they developed professionally in an era where microaggressions and discriminatory behaviors were often tolerated as way of survival (Iheduru-Anderson et al., 2022). This "survival mode" may have blinded the mentor's own experiences with and recollection of discrimination during their time as a student, making it difficult for mentors to discern their mentees' experiences with microaggression as racism versus a general culture in nursing education that supports incivility (Eka & Chambers, 2019). Further, mentors' own success in overcoming challenges based on their racial/ethnic identity may dissuade them from encouraging anti-racism behaviors among their mentees.

The work of being anti-racist takes a toll on resources for both the students and their mentors, and often places the onus on the victim. For example, because some forms of racially and ethnically based aggressions are often not recognized by the person committing the acts (e.g., behaviors resulting from implicit bias), the recipient of that act often carries the responsibility of calling it out. While this may be accomplished with a simple anti-racist strategy such as asking a clarifying question, as anti-racist responses from schools of nursing become more robust, they often result in multiple facilitated meetings to create awareness about the situation and, at times, resolve the conflict. This is a difficult emotional process for all involved that may have particularly devastating effects for minoritized nursing students and their mentors, who may have experienced a history of racial/ethnically based aggressions and other intersecting traumas and may ultimately interfere with academic performance and productivity.

Necessary transformation in the policies, practices, and cultures of schools of nursing will be essential to truly support mentoring of minoritized nursing students to promote anti-racism. First, it is critical that minoritized students and their mentors do not take the sole responsibility of this work. Improving awareness of these issues and providing anti-racist bystander training is critical. In doing so, it is important to consider this as an ongoing process that includes comprehensive and ongoing training that is not just one time. Second, schools of nursing should recognize the added "diversity tax" that racial/ethnic minoritized mentors play in supporting their students. In doing so, it is important to consider the added time and resource investment required in effective mentoring and support of minoritized students in workload assignments. Third, schools of nursing need to ensure that resources are available to support minoritized students and their mentors and that these resources take on a trauma-informed approach that considers any anti-racist act within the context of a history of racialized traumas that may intersect with other experiences (e.g., adverse childhood experiences). Finally, leaders with diverse identities, especially the white majority, are needed to serve as champions of anti-racism, promoting a culture that provides positive reinforcement when incidents are called out and ensuring that the burden is not placed on individuals who are most likely to have experienced aggressions and traumas in the past.

Transformations to support mentoring minoritized nursing students to promote anti-racism:

1. Minoritized nursing students and mentors should not take sole responsibility for promoting anti-racism.
2. The "diversity tax" experienced by minoritized mentors should be recognized.
3. Schools of nursing need to provide trauma-informed resources to support minoritized students and mentors.
4. Leaders with diverse identities need to serve as champions of anti-racism.

References

Bell, B. (2021). White dominance in nursing education: A target for anti-racist efforts. *Nursing Inquiry, 28*(1), e12379. https://doi.org/10.1111/nin.12379

Cary, M. P., Randolph, S. D., Broome, M. E., & Carter, B. M. (2020). Creating a culture that values diversity and inclusion: An action-oriented framework for schools of nursing. *Nursing Forum, 55*(4), 687–694. https://doi.org/10.1111/nuf.12485

Coleman, T. (2020). Anti-racism in nursing education: Recommendations for racial justice praxis. *Journal of Nursing Education, 59*(11), 642–645. https://doi.org/10.3928/01484834-20201020-08

Eka, N. G. A., & Chambers, D. (2019). Incivility in nursing education: A systematic literature review. *Nurse Education in Practice, 39*, 45–54. doi: 10.1016/j.nepr.2019.06.004

Elias, A., Ben, J., Mansouri, F., & Paradies, Y. (2021). Racism and nationalism during and beyond the COVID-19 pandemic. *Ethnic and Racial Studies, 44*(5), 783–793. https://doi.org/10.1080/01419870.2020.1851382

Iheduru-Anderson, K., Okoro, F. O., & Moore, S. S. (2022). Diversity and inclusion or tokens? A qualitative study of Black women academic nurse leaders in the United States. *Global Qualitative Nursing Research, 9.* https://doi.org/10.1177/23333936211073116

Mackey, K., Ayers, C. K., Kondo, K. K., Saha, S., Advani, S. M., Young, S., Spencer, H., Rusek, M., Anderson, J., Veazie, S., Smith, M., & Kansagara, D. (2021). Racial and ethnic disparities in COVID-19–related infections, hospitalizations, and deaths: A systematic review. *Annals of Internal Medicine, 174*(3), 362–373. https://doi.org/10.7326/M20-6306

Mendenhall, E., Kohrt, B. A., Logie, C. H., & Tsai, A. C. (2022). Syndemics and clinical science. *Nature Medicine, 28*(7), 1359–1362. https://doi.org/10.1038/s41591-022-01888-y

National Academies of Sciences, Engineering, and Medicine. (2020). *The science of effective mentorship in STEMM.* https://www.nationalacademies.org/our-work/the-science-of-effective-mentoring-in-stemm

Osakwe, Z. T., Obioha, C. U., Minuti, A., Atairu, M., & Osborne, J. C. (2022). Barriers and facilitators to success in undergraduate nursing education among minority students. *Nurse Educator*, published ahead of print. https://doi.org/10.1097/nne.0000000000001154

Wilson, F. A., & Stimpson, J. P. (2020). US policies increase vulnerability of immigrant communities to the COVID-19 pandemic. *Annals of Global Health, 86*(1), 57. http://doi.org/10.5334/aogh.2897

Now, More Than Ever, Diversity Matters

Gaurdia Banister, PhD, RN, NEA-BC, FAAN
Executive Director of the Institute for Patient Care, Massachusetts General Hospital

When you're the "only one" for so much of your life, you grow up wanting things to be different. I grew up in Casper, Wyoming, where the Black population was less than 1% (State of Wyoming, n.d.). My parents had moved there in 1957 from New Orleans, a place where racism and discrimination were woven into the fabric of daily living in the city. They wanted a better life, better schools, and better opportunities for themselves, my brother, and me. They certainly succeeded, and I am grateful for their courage to make such a radical change in our lives. However, I experienced an isolation and loneliness that is hard to explain. Sometimes I wonder how I got through it all.

As I look back on my nursing career, I was the only African American in my school of nursing class. I had only one African American teacher throughout my entire education, from grade school through undergraduate and graduate nursing education. I am grateful that I didn't get the messages that some acquaintances and friends would receive in their nursing programs and academic careers. I would hear stories about the challenges faced by students of color as they tried to become nurses. Comments ranged from "you aren't smart enough" to "I'm really not sure this profession is for you," and much more. These messages had a devastating impact on many of my friends. Some persevered and made it through; others did not.

> "The capability to be inclusive largely defines us, and holding multiple perspectives without judgment is the essence of putting it on public display. Mentoring is the tilling of the soil by which the implicit is made explicit and all can flourish. Together this understanding and these acts not only bend the arc of health equity but also catalyze the necessary movement of rhetoric into reality through ways of being, knowing, storytelling, and the authentic sharing of the self."
>
> –G. Rumay Alexander, EdD, RN, FAAN
> Professor, University of North Carolina School of Nursing

This background served as a foundation and catalyst (and ignited my passion) for advancing diversity and inclusion as a nurse leader in the profession of nursing. Developing a pipeline for diverse nurses to succeed in my profession fueled my soul. I promised myself that things would be different—something had to be different. I didn't know how or when or how it would happen, but I knew or hoped I would make a difference. All this has been reinforced in texts such as *The Future of Nursing 2020–2030: Charting a Path to Achieve Health Equity* (National Academies of Sciences, Engineering, and Medicine, 2021).

While I have proudly served as a mentor and preceptor for many diverse nurses throughout the years, it became clear that some students and nurses of color, in general, may need more help and support. I also learned that one-on-one interactions between students of color and practitioners of color could be transformative. Establishing systems and models to advance diversity and inclusion can create sustainable change and greater impact. Furthermore, community and educational partnerships are essential and the key to success.

Two programs in which I assumed a leadership role serve as models to advance diversity in nursing and have special meaning to me. The first is the Health Alliance: Creating Workforce Diversity program, which received federal funding when I was a Senior Vice President and CNO at Providence Hospital in Washington, DC. Providence Hospital is a community hospital committed to providing exemplary healthcare to the community that addressed the needs of the marginalized and disenfranchised who sought care. We partnered with the local community college, the University of the District of Columbia, and the Urban Alliance in this program. They worked with schools and employers, such as our hospital, to address systemic barriers to economic mobility for young adults of color and to bridge the gaps between education and workforce development.

This project aimed to develop and implement a program that would prepare and support disadvantaged and minoritized high school graduates interested in a career in nursing to enter and successfully complete an associate degree program in nursing. The project's overall goal was to provide the pathway and support for students to complete a nursing education program and begin work as registered nurses in the District of Columbia. We knew that helping these young women (we had no men at the time) who desperately wanted to become nurses realize their dreams would change the trajectory of their lives and the lives of their families; they would serve as role models for others who aspired for more. An additional feature of the Health Alliance program was attention to social needs and challenges.

A second program, the Clinical Leadership Collaborative for Diversity in Nursing, is another workforce development model designed to achieve, in part, the vision of increasing diversity in nursing by facilitating the successful progression of socioeconomically disadvantaged students through the generic undergraduate nursing program at the University of Massachusetts, Boston, College of Nursing and Health Sciences (Banister et al., 2014; Banister & Winfrey, 2012). This program is funded by the Mass General Brigham Health Care system. Under the leadership of Jeanette Ives Erickson, our chief nurse council recognized a desperate need to attract and retain a more diverse nursing workforce if we genuinely wanted to deliver exemplary care.

Both programs included scholarship support, stipends for living expenses, professional development activities, tutoring, National Council Licensure Examination preparation, pairing students with nurse mentors for coaching and support, educational opportunities, and priority for clinical placements and ultimately employment post-graduation.

In closing, close to 250 students participated and graduated from the programs, and here are a couple of quotes from the graduates:

> "I'm evolving more into an advocate for people who don't have voices, because I realize I was given a platform and that should be of benefit to other people."

> "It wasn't just like, here's just money to get through this college. It was just like, here are the people who want to see you do better, and here are the people who are going through what you're going through. You know when you have people telling you here are the resources for you to do well and for you to become successful, it's just kind of like, all right, I'm going to be successful, I'm going to do this, I'm going to try hard . . . I felt[it] was powerful."

There is undoubtedly more work to do, but I'm proud to be part of the process to diversify our profession! I hope no student or nurse ever has to feel like I felt again.

References

Banister, G., Bowen-Brady, H., & Winfrey, M. E. (2014). Using career nurse mentors to support minority nursing students and facilitate their transition to practice. *Journal of Professional Nursing, 30*(4), 317–325.

Banister, G., & Winfrey, M. E. (2012). Enhancing diversity in nursing, a partnership approach. *Journal of Nursing Administration, 42*(3), 176–181.

National Academies of Sciences, Engineering, and Medicine. (2021). *The future of nursing 2020–2030: Charting a path to achieve health equity.* National Academies Press. https://nam.edu/publications/the-future-of-nursing-2020-2030

State of Wyoming. (n.d.). *Demographic profiles for Wyoming and counties: 1970.* http://eadiv.state.wy.us/demog_data/pop1970/

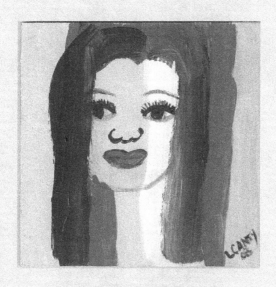

IN THE SHADOWS

I have been living in a shadow of a doubt
People questioning my existence
Wondering who, why, how did I get here
Trying to understand why someone like me
Black and female
Was able to survive years of oppression
Years of being held back
How could I be motivated to move beyond
What society deemed to be my future
In the shadows, I would receive guidance
Love and support
In the shadow, would be where I learned my history
Where I would understand my past
Where I would feel how my ancestors influenced my present
In the shadows, I would learn how to love myself
And appreciate what I had to offer
Without a shadow of a doubt
I know I have a right to be here

Poetry and artwork by Lucinda Canty, PhD, CNM, FACNM
Associate Professor of Nursing, University of Massachusetts Amherst

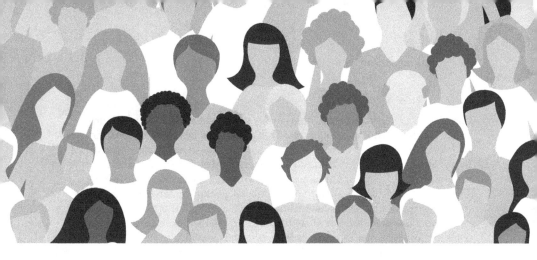

4 Care Delivery: Quality, Safety, Access

In This Chapter

- Health-Related Social Needs: Acknowledging and Impacting National Inequities

- A Personal Journey to Improving Maternal Health

- Addressing the Crack in the Healthcare Foundation

- Improving Healthcare by Meeting People Where They Are

- Harnessing the Power of Nursing to Improve Care Delivery for Marginalized Populations

Care delivery includes access to high-quality, consistent healthcare, which promotes health equity. Expanding care delivery to serve minoritized and marginalized populations whenever, wherever, and however they need care is also essential for fostering health equity. Nurses must remember that during our interactions with those we serve, we are often presented with only a snapshot of their life. Therefore, care delivery must be nonjudgmental, person-centered, and considerate of sociocultural factors and identities that may preclude optimal health outcomes. For some, this may mean thinking outside the box or getting out of one's comfort zone, but to ensure that healthcare is provided to all in an equitable manner, nurses must go beyond what is comfortable and what may be the traditional, standard route to provide the healthcare that is needed for each patient or client to maximize their opportunity to be healthy.

Consider the following questions as you read the essays about health equity and care delivery:

- What steps can be taken to address social determinants of health through healthcare delivery?

- How can the community or community members be involved in improving outcomes of marginalized populations?

- What role do nurses play in finding solutions to historical issues that have led to health inequities?

- How can nurses' delivery of healthcare support at-risk and marginalized populations to promote health equity?

- What are examples of how nurses have been innovative with healthcare delivery?

Health-Related Social Needs: Acknowledging and Impacting National Inequities

Cyrus Batheja, EdD, MBA, BSN, RN, PHN, FAAN
National Vice President, Enterprise Transformation and Strategic Solutions,
UnitedHealthcare

Treyce Gladney, MBA
Director of Health Equity and Strategy, UnitedHealthcare

Growing up as a first-generation immigrant in a single-parent household that barely had money to pay rent and keep food on the table, healthcare was viewed as a luxury that was only accessed on an as-needed basis. These experiences shaped my views on healthcare. My understanding of healthcare shifted only after my family progressed up the socioeconomic ladder. I began to understand and appreciate the importance of preventive health and the value of nutrition and exercise. The research underlines that our lived experiences shape how we understand and engage our health (Daines et al., 2021). Moreover, barriers to essential needs like food, transportation, housing, employment, and access to care profoundly impact our health and well-being. People who encounter difficulties with basic social needs have less ability to achieve optimal well-being.

> *"Each patient added to a hospital staff nurse's workload is associated with a 7 to 12% increase in mortality as well as significantly lower patient and nurse satisfaction. Each 10% increase in the proportion of hospital staff nurses with bachelor's degrees is associated with a 7% decline in patient mortality. Evidence-based nurse staffing, a bachelor's qualified nurse workforce, and supportive work environments save lives and money and retain great nurses in clinical care."*
>
> –Linda H. Aiken, PhD, RN, FAAN, FRCN
> Professor of Nursing and Sociology
> Founding Director, Center for Health Outcomes and Policy Research
> University of Pennsylvania

Addressing a person's social barriers is imperative to improving their overall health and well-being. Acknowledging the challenges outlined above, I joined UnitedHealthcare, a division of UnitedHealth Group, a diversified health and well-being company with a mission to help people live healthier lives and help make the health system work better for everyone. Together, with a team focused on addressing the social determinants of health (SDOH) that includes my co-author, Treyce Gladney, we aim to:

1. Learn about social barriers by screening

2. Address the social needs identified through our screening

3. Follow up with members who received our support to identify if their needs were met or not

4. Escalate all unmet member needs to a team focused on addressing these challenges

5. Produce analytics to understand the impact on members and communities

Intentional screening is the foundation for learning about our members' social barriers. Our approach to screening includes both evaluation and survey. United-Healthcare considers the member at the center of our actions. Our member-centered design allows us to consider the unique barriers faced by different groups of people before the screening. To address SDOH, we design outreach activities using a health equity lens, assessing the impact on historically marginalized groups before engaging them. The questions we use in surveys are evidence-based and concise; when we identify needs, we provide prompt support and follow-up to determine if needs were met.

Our screening questions leverage simple, intentional statements customized to the surveyed population. We seek to understand our members' unique needs, identify gaps, and deliver tailored solutions to advance health equity. We use empathy as a bridge to building authentic, healing relationships and uncovering health inequities rooted in lived experiences. In our model, we carefully craft questions by thoughtfully selecting each word and aligning them to the professional delivering the survey. We recognize our members' ethos and that there are limited opportunities to interact with them to fully understand their situations. We value their time and avoid conflating multiple questions into one, considering what can be actionable.

We recognize there are limitations to the types of impacts produced by referring people to community resources; however, our screening questions are action-oriented, creating connections between a member's responses and available resources within their community. In partnership with community-based organization aggregators, we procure systems that allow us to see community resource availability and ensure that there are adequate resources to support when members prompt having a need. These systems also provide us with active feedback on whether a member's needs were met or not. One example of how we tie all these elements together at UnitedHealthcare is through the deployment of a national community health worker (CHW) model. Inside UnitedHealthcare's SDOH program, the role of CHWs is unique because of their ability to develop trusting relationships with populations that have greater social and health needs than average. Our CHW model leverages lay people from the community and peers with a shared sense of identity. Our field-based staff can relate to lived experience and demonstrate a working knowledge of the community. They serve as an essential liaison between the community, medical, and public health systems.

How the UnitedHealthcare CHW Initiative Got Started

In 2019, just before the COVID-19 pandemic hit, our organization was challenged to build a program to recognize the social needs of our members and address inequities within the communities we serve. Understanding that members with complex social needs require more robust support, we developed a CHW program, hiring people from the community to help our members. Our CHWs work telephonically and face to face; they are trained to guide and motivate members using trauma-informed care and motivational interviewing. The teams help identify barriers to appropriate care and create action plans with members to improve access and adherence. Importantly, this provides our national teams qualitative insights to better understand community-based inequities, which we leverage while developing strategic initiatives to remove barriers to health.

The CHW model that emerged had an underlying plan to make an impact in the local community. As the team crafted the blueprint for aligning organizational resources to screen and engage members in meeting their basic social needs, it sparked a desire to build a deeper community connection centered on meaningfully addressing inequities in our communities. This alignment of addressing social needs and equity simultaneously became critical, especially as we looked to activate historically marginalized communities. There is an interconnection between leveraging lived experiences and application to screening using a health equity lens. The connections go beyond screening and raise the question of training that allows for a tactic to help us understand how others are feeling so we can respond appropriately to the situation or, as the definition applies, with empathy. Barriers to essential needs like food, transportation, housing, employment, and access to financial tools profoundly impact our health and well-being. The authors and their teams are actively working to continue responding to members who encounter difficulties accessing their basic social needs to improve their overall health.

Reference

Daines, C. L., Hansen, D., Novilla, M. L. B., & Crandall, A. (2021). Effects of positive and negative childhood experiences on adult family health. *BMC Public Health*, 21(651). https://doi.org/10.1186/s12889-021-10732-w

A Personal Journey to Improving Maternal Health

Cynthia Barginere, DNP, RN, FACHE
Chief Operating Officer, Institute for Healthcare Improvement

My mother didn't have her first pregnancy until her late 30s. She experienced a full-term pregnancy, but her first child, Robert, was stillborn. She talked about the experience of having Robert for most of my childhood. She shared the difficulty of her labor. She described how no one paid attention when she tried to say, "Something doesn't feel right." She expressed the pain of delivering a baby that was dead and not having the opportunity to really say goodbye. Understandably, my mother's view of childbirth was filled with pain and fear. I used to muse that maybe her stories were meant as a method of birth control for me, her oldest daughter. But as I got older and learned of the risks to older pregnant people, and particularly Black people, I came to understand her fears. And to share them.

My early career as an Intensive Care Unit (ICU) nurse only increased my worries. All my experiences with childbirth in the ICU ended in tragedy. I saw too many young Black women admitted with strokes, too many women who had stillbirths. Then, at 24, I became pregnant. When I told my mother I had big news, she was not happy. Her first words were, "Please don't tell me you are pregnant." When I called with the news of my second pregnancy, she said, "Please don't tell me you are pregnant again." I didn't understand her lack of excitement. I knew her feelings about her own pregnancy, but I expected her to be thrilled about the prospect of grandchildren.

My first pregnancy ended in miscarriage. When I got pregnant again, I started to better understand my mother's feelings. I took on her fears. I was afraid of another miscarriage. I was afraid of stillbirth, stroke, pain. Yet even my own experiences and those of my mother were not enough to help me fully understand the risks of pregnancy for Black birthing people. It took working with colleagues in obstetrics when I was the Chief Nursing Officer and Associate Executive Director for the Women & Children's Division at the University of Alabama at Birmingham (UAB) for me to see the bigger picture.

The US has consistently demonstrated a higher maternal mortality rate than other developed countries, with Black and Hispanic women faring worse than their white counterparts. According to the February 2022 report from the National Center for Health Statistics (2022), there was an increase in the absolute number of maternal deaths and in the number of deaths per 1,000 live births from 2019 to 2020. The report showed the maternal mortality rate for Black women was 2.9 times the rate for white women.

At UAB, I saw the number of women who came to the hospital without having received adequate (or any) prenatal care when they were either in crisis or at the point of delivery. In partnership with UAB's Chair of Obstetrics & Gynecology, we created targeted interventions to support at-risk pregnant people in the region. In collaboration with the Jefferson County Department of Public Health (DPH), we placed obstetrics residents and nurse practitioners in DPH offices in rural and low-population areas to provide prenatal care for pregnant people at risk of morbidity, mortality, or premature delivery. We encouraged the moms with then innovative 3D ultrasounds and the choice of a free car seat or breast pump (to encourage breastfeeding) upon discharge. We designed an Obstetrics Emergency Service to care for every pregnant woman. We provided needed care and services to high-risk pregnant people and, as a result, saw a significant increase in delivery volume.

Years later, when I worked in a tertiary care center in Alabama, I again saw the trend of birthing people with high-risk pregnancies visiting the emergency department and delivering without having had the advantage of prenatal care. I worked closely with maternal fetal medicine physicians and the Alabama Medicaid Agency to implement a Centering Pregnancy program, a patient-centered model that provides group prenatal care. The program demonstrated decreased rates of preterm and low-birth-weight babies and increased breastfeeding rates.

Today, I am proud to work as Chief Operating Officer at the Institute for Healthcare Improvement (IHI). IHI is committed to equitably improving maternal health and reducing maternal deaths across the globe. I am privileged to continue the work that honors my mother and the brother I never had the opportunity to know.

Reference

National Center for Health Statistics. (2022). *Maternal mortality rates in the United States, 2020.* https://www.cdc.gov/nchs/data/hestat/maternal-mortality/2020/e-stat-maternal-mortality-rates-2022.pdf

Addressing the Crack in the Healthcare Foundation

Sarah L. Szanton, PhD, RN, FAAN
Dean & Patricia M. Davidson Health Equity and Social Justice Endowed Professor
Johns Hopkins School of Nursing

The most compelling levers for equity are those that are universally recognizable. In an ideal world, this might look like seeing each human as worthy of dignity or addressing our country's sins of enslavement of people and theft of lands and traditions from the original inhabitants. But in a world where people do not share core values, it is useful to think through the lens of others and consider more practical reasons to address dignity, justice, and equity for all. As Isabel Wilkerson in her book *Caste* (2020) observes: She couldn't avoid fixing the cracked foundation of her house just because neither she nor her ancestors had initially built the house. Whether she caused the foundation to crack or not, it required a solution. Similarly, we may not all agree, but we do all live in a country with a cracked foundation, and all of us have a role in its repair.

I was a health policy advocate prior to coming to nursing. Partly due to this experience, in my research career I have used improving the function of older adults as a pathway to the pursuit of equity. Aging should be universally invested in. If we are lucky, all of us will age. But beyond that view, because older adults with functional limitations cost two to three times more to Medicaid and Medicare than older adults without these functional limitations, even people who do not necessarily care about equity can see the fiscal benefit in addressing function among older adults (Wolff et al., 2019). Due to these facts, and to insights from clinical experiences providing house calls to homebound adults, I co-developed the CAPABLE program to help older adults achieve equity in independence and to save money for society.

CAPABLE is a four to five month, participant-directed, home-based program that increases mobility and function of older adults in their home environment. CAPABLE achieves this through identifying what matters to the older adult, their strengths and home environment, and tailoring the program specifically to those goals. An interprofessional team comprised of an occupational therapist (OT) and an RN work with the older adult to understand the person's goals (e.g., to walk downstairs, take a shower, and get dressed without pain), and then use modern behavioral science, such as action planning, along with the work of a handyman, to enable the older adult to achieve them. In the CAPABLE program, the team conducts 10 in-home visits with participants to achieve the six patient-centered functional goals the older adult has set.

As examples, if a participant wants to prepare food rather than wait for a neighbor to help, the OT and participant strategize feasible energy-conserving approaches and tools. To complement these strategies, the nurse uses behavioral activation strategies to help the participant manage depressive symptoms and balance issues. And the handyman stabilizes stairs, levels flooring, and repairs floors to enable participants to practice newly learned mobility skills safely and efficiently.

Multiple peer-reviewed studies show that CAPABLE reduces disability, reduces depressive symptoms, increases falls self-efficacy (confidence in completing activities of daily living without falling), and reduces costs through reduced hospitalizations and nursing home visits (savings of approximately $22,000 per participant over two years; Ruiz et al., 2017; Szanton et al., 2021). CAPABLE participants routinely describe the life-changing impact of newly being able to take a bath, cook a meal with ease, or go to community events.

CAPABLE is an equity approach because it is tailored to each individual's strengths and goals. The clinicians do not presuppose anyone's goals nor their individual strengths. In CAPABLE, each person gets the same number of visits and potential goals, but the program completely tailors the content to each older adult. One person's goals may be to make meals without pain and shortness of breath, while another's might be to walk down the stairs and get into a car.

As is the case for CAPABLE, nurses have a place in securing equity for the communities they serve. Nurses understand the context of daily life and how that interacts with all the other aspects of health and life. As a profession, our impact is muted until we persuade policymakers of the population health impact of an equitable approach. Nurses have vital training and perspective in devising solutions that are equitable and tailored to individual or populations' needs. But we must go beyond our own work and values to think creatively and through the lenses of multiple layers of stakeholders to be able to move equity forward. What is important to us may not be immediately important to someone else. We will need to listen, to speak the language of policy and business, to understand others' points of view, and then detail the ways our solution will be beneficial to everyone.

As the future of nursing report makes clear, nursing must work to achieve health equity "built on strengthened nursing capacity and expertise" (National Academies of Sciences, Engineering, and Medicine et al., 2021, p. 1). We are perfectly positioned to bring together public health, healthcare, social services, and public policy. But we will also need to flourish in the population health work that pays for health outcomes and wellness above patient visits. As the fiscal incentives align with population health, we will be there to lead and to ensure that the people we serve of all backgrounds and health states are included in equity solutions. Showing the health, fiscal, and political benefits for our patients, stakeholders, and decision-makers will help enable this.

CAPABLE is one model where this is proving to be successful. And it can be a model for other nursing and public health nursing and interdisciplinary team efforts to meet each person where they are, both literally and metaphorically.

Physical and cognitive function are some of the keys to equity. There are so many population health areas that nurses lead, such as children's health, parenting, mental health, reproductive health, infectious disease, and others. Our nation's health will be served as nursing rises to the grand challenge of devising equity solutions for all and communicating them into policy change.

References

National Academies of Sciences, Engineering, and Medicine. (2021). *The future of nursing 2020–2030: Charting a path to achieve health equity*. National Academies Press. https://nam.edu/publications/the-future-of-nursing-2020-2030

Ruiz, S., Snyder, L. P., Rotondo, C., Cross-Barnet, C., Colligan, E. M., & Giuriceo, K. (2017). Innovative home visit models associated with reductions in costs, hospitalizations, and emergency department use. *Health Affairs, 36*(3), 425–432. https://doi.org/10.1377/hlthaff.2016.1305

Szanton, S. L., Leff, B., Li, Q., Breysse, J., Spoelstra, S., Kell, J., Purvis, J., Xue, Q., Wilson, J., & Gitlin, L. N. (2021). CAPABLE program improves disability in multiple randomized trials. *Journal of the American Geriatrics Society, 69*(12), 3631–3640. https://doi.org/10.1111/jgs.17383

Wilkerson, I. (2020). *Caste: The origins of our discontents*. Random House.

Wolff, J., Nicholas, L. H., Willink, A., Mulcahy, J., Davis, K., & Kasper, J. (2019). *Not receiving needed help with daily activities may increase Medicare spending*. The Commonwealth Fund. https://www.commonwealthfund.org/publications/journal-article/2019/jun/not-receiving-needed-help-may-increase-medicare-spending

Improving Healthcare by Meeting People Where They Are

Julius Johnson, DNP, FNP-BC, FAANP
Department Chair
School of Nursing at Long Island University Brooklyn

Carter Todd, MS, MBA, RN, CCRN
Assistant Nurse Manager, Kaiser Permanente

When you picture a nurse in your mind, who do you see? Historically speaking, the nurse persona was reserved for white bonnet caps with finely pressed dresses. Our experience as registered nurses has served as a juxtaposition of the common narrative in both healthcare and society. Practicing the art and science of nursing in the acute care setting helped us realize that our profession was gifted with the scope, duty, and heart to be the glue holding the healthcare industry together. Nurses make up the largest segment in the healthcare professions, allowing for our abilities to spill out from hospital walls and over into our neighborhoods and school districts. We have built our practice from a deeply rooted appreciation for the responsibility we have to our community as compassionate healthcare professionals who really understand people. Nursing is the touchpoint on the end of healthcare's fingertips, reaching out to the community while being able to speak all languages and connect with all of America's backgrounds.

> *"Care delivery as a registered nurse is the most significant work you can do, instilling a sense of pride through proper staffing levels and inspirational nursing leadership designed for the perfect work environment for patients to thrive, families to feel confident, and clinicians to request their desired unit by name."*
>
> –P. K. Scheerle, RN
> CEO Emeritus, Gifted Healthcare

To overcome the deep, historical mistrust of the healthcare system within the Black community and create vaccine equity during the COVID-19 pandemic, we had to reimagine and redesign the way that the Black community experienced the healthcare system. The first step was to deliver the care in a safe space that was also highly trusted in the Black community. One of the most trusted places within Black communities is the Black church. We decided to create a standing clinic within a Black church in the east New York neighborhood of Brooklyn. The second part of the redesign was to staff the site with providers that reflected the culture of the targeted audience. This led to a partnership between a community health center (Community Health Network) and the Greater NYC Black Nurses Association (GNYCBNA). The last step was assuring that the providers and community partners were thoroughly prepared to handle the volume of people attending the vaccine clinic while also being willing to understand the hesitancy people would have as they came into the clinic. The result of this collaboration and redesigning of healthcare delivery was a culturally competent vaccine clinic. The African American and other residents of the borough gave the providers very high satisfaction results for their work within the clinic. It was so successful that the clinic design was duplicated within Jamaica, Queens, and led to more than 60 vaccine pop-up clinics. In the end we distributed over 30,000 vaccines, and more than 70% of those vaccines were given to Black and Latinx members of the community. This innovative collaboration and design directly resulted in the creation of vaccine equity in some communities.

Owning our narrative as Black men in nursing creates a pathway to be seen for the historically unseen Black man's health status. As nurses of color, owning the narrative has been a challenge met with perseverance and collaboration. Being leaders both locally and nationally within the National Black Nurses Association, we are afforded a platform to own the narrative of who the nurse persona could be for the people in our communities. While in graduate school, Carter conducted research for his thesis work, *A Qualitative Study of the African American Man's Perception of Nursing as a Career: Barbershop Talk*, with the aim of bridging the gap between healthcare and the Black male community through honest, open, authentic dialogue with people in a comfortable and relatable atmosphere (Todd, 2019). This graduate work has continued on several years later with new and improved iterations to bridge the gap.

The model of barbershop health outreach is one that has been used before. Our success in barbershop health promotion stems from using our nursing skill set to navigate an environment in which we are uniquely positioned to succeed. We learned that being ourselves, above all else, was the key to our success. Being young healthcare professionals who can navigate multiple different social arenas flips on its head the constraints of who Black men are allowed and expected to be in our country. We diverge from the socialized expectations of a compassionate and trusted touch from a nurse being expected only in the hospital setting. The dichotomy of these different worlds is melded together with outreach programs focused on the barbershop. We know Black men fare far worse in life expectancy than other groups, so why not meet our people where they are and arm ourselves with discussions that promote health literacy? Aligning with evidence concluding that increased nurse staffing in hospitals lowers mortality (Aiken et al., 2018), we believe that same postulation holds true in the community setting, where more nurses in any community will directly correlate to improved healthcare outcomes.

Another example of redesigning healthcare to increase the delivery of interventions to marginalized populations was the creation of Last Night a DJ Saved My Life Alliance. This alliance is a partnership between a world class DJ, a local nurse, and GNYCBNA. GNYCBNA created an opioid overdose prevention program under the NYC Department of Health and began going into the community to train community members on how to recognize signs of overdosing and how to administer Narcan safely. DJ Lauren Flax took the initiative to new heights when she collaborated with GNYCBNA and took the trainings to nightclubs. Although drug use is often seen as taboo, a place with known frequent drug use is nightclubs. Instead of approaching it as taboo, the collaboration directly trained staff, including bartenders, security guards, and owners, on how to administer Narcan to their nightclub patrons. This led to an increased amount of Narcan being available during times that marginalized populations may have needed to utilize it. This innovative design increased the demand for Narcan trainings throughout NYC nightlife.

These examples illustrate the innovative and culturally competent methods needed to address care delivery in the community, which is extremely important for reducing health disparities in minoritized and other underserved populations.

Reference

Aiken, L. H., Cerón, C., Simonetti, M., Lake, E. T., Galiano, A., Garbarini, A., Soto, P., Bravo, D., & Smith, H. L. (2018). Hospital nurse staffing and patient outcomes. *Revista Médica Clínica Las Condes, 29*(3), 322–327. https://doi.org/10.1016/j.rmclc.2018.04.011

Todd, C. (2019). *A qualitative study of the African American man's perception of nursing as a career: Barbershop talk.* (Publication No. 22617052) [Master's thesis, University of California Davis]. ProQuest Dissertations Publishing

Harnessing the Power of Nursing to Improve Care Delivery for Marginalized Populations

Billy A. Caceres, PhD, RN, FAHA, FAAN
Assistant Professor of Nursing
Columbia University School of Nursing

Over the past decade, there has been increasing attention to the impact that social determinants have on driving population health (National Academies of Sciences, Engineering, and Medicine, 2021; National Advisory Council on Nurse Education and Practice, 2020). Many of the health and healthcare disparities that have been documented in the United States and globally are largely attributed to social determinants of health (such as poverty, neighborhood and built environment, and limited access to needed healthcare services). For instance, researchers have found that social determinants predict hospital readmissions among marginalized populations (including older and low-income adults; Buitrago et al., 2021; Zhang et al., 2020). The COVID-19 pandemic has shone a spotlight on the inequities that exist within our healthcare system (Russo et al., 2021), economic and healthcare systems in the United States, and the burden of disease associated with social determinants of health (SDOH). Yet, nurses and other healthcare professionals receive very little education on the role of social determinants in shaping population health. And they often lack the resources to appropriately address these major contributors to health outcomes. These factors limit our profession's ability to make meaningful and sustained changes to improve the health of our patients.

My research program focuses on understanding and addressing social determinants of cardiovascular health in marginalized populations with a focus on lesbian, gay, bisexual, transgender, and queer (LGBTQ+) and racial and ethnic minoritized populations. I was inspired to conduct this research based on my experiences caring for cardiothoracic and vascular surgery patients at various hospitals in New

York City. As a clinical nurse, I witnessed firsthand that much of what determined health outcomes for my patients was related to factors that we had little control over as nurses in the hospital setting. I quickly realized that social determinants including, but not limited to, social isolation, inability to pay for medications, housing and food insecurity, and low health literacy were major contributors to hospital readmissions and negative health outcomes following surgical procedures. Despite working at world-class institutions, I often felt powerless and incapable of helping my patients that were most in need. Simply telling my patients what they needed to do to improve their health could only go so far because I was rarely able to help them address the root causes of the health problems they were experiencing.

As we gain a greater understanding that social determinants of health are important drivers of health and healthcare disparities, it is crucial for nurses across all settings to be equipped with the tools to appropriately address these. As a profession, we need to recognize and appreciate that what happens outside the walls of clinics and hospitals is just as important (and I argue often more important) as what happens during healthcare encounters. To truly make a difference in the health of marginalized populations, our profession needs to adopt approaches that reimagine healthcare delivery to fully harness the power of nursing to eliminate health and healthcare disparities.

The continued persistence of health and healthcare disparities suggests that existing models of healthcare delivery are not sufficient to bring about health equity. For example, within cardiovascular health research, my area of expertise, there have been numerous behavioral interventions to reduce cardiovascular disease risk in Black and Latinx adults (Estrada et al., 2021; White et al., 2020), the fastest growing ethnic minoritized group in the United States, are at a high risk for cardiovascular disease (CVD). However, the majority of these interventions have had limited effectiveness at bringing about sustained improvements in the cardiovascular health of these marginalized populations. Very few of these interventions target social determinants of health (such as discrimination and neighborhood environment) to improve the cardiovascular health of these groups.

We cannot talk about delivery of nursing care without addressing other areas of nursing. In the following sections I provide my top recommendations for nurse leaders and nurses to improve care delivery for marginalized populations.

Recommendations for Nursing Practice

- Develop new nurse-led interprofessional models of care in hospital and community settings to comprehensively address social determinants of health.

- Collaborate with experts outside of healthcare (such as urban planners, architects, and engineers) to address ways in which our built environments can be redesigned to optimize health and well-being.

- Ensure that nurses across practice settings understand the role of social determinants in shaping health outcomes.

Recommendations for Nursing Research

- Call for increased funding for research projects that support collaboration between nurse scientists and community-based organizations to address the most pressing health concerns in low-income and other underserved communities.

- Develop and test multi-level interventions to address social determinants of health.

- Incorporate measurement of social determinants of health as common data elements in nursing research.

Recommendations for Policy

- Partner with lawmakers and other stakeholders to support policies that address root causes of health and healthcare disparities (such as income inequality).

- Advocate for greater funding for demonstration projects that test novel nurse-led models of care delivery that target potentially modifiable social determinants of health (such as loneliness and food insecurity).

Recommendations for Nursing Education

- Educate nursing students that social determinants (such as racism), not social identities (such as race and ethnicity), are the causes of health and healthcare disparities.

- Integrate content about social determinants and social justice across courses in pre-licensure and graduate nursing programs. Discussion of these important concepts should not be limited only to public health nursing courses.

- Partner with community-based organizations to provide greater opportunities for pre-licensure students to complete student nurse externships in community settings.

- Increase investments in programs to diversify nursing student bodies and nurse faculty.

Despite all the work that is needed in our profession to ensure that healthcare delivery truly addresses the needs of our most marginalized patient populations, this is an exciting time in nursing. We are now having more open conversations about the ways in which our profession has previously failed those most in need. We must also do more to diversify our profession so that nurses reflect the diversity of our patient populations. Although often painful, confronting these harsh realities is needed to redesign the way in which we conceptualize and deliver nursing care and to guarantee that the voices of those that have long been ignored are heard, valued, and acknowledged.

References

Buitrago, I., Seidl, K. L., Gingold, D. B., & Marcozzi, D. (2021). Analysis of readmissions in a mobile integrated health transitional care program using root cause analysis and common cause analysis. *Journal for Healthcare Quality*. Advance online publication. https://doi.org/10.1097/JHQ.0000000000000328

Estrada, L. V., Solano, J., Reading Turchioe, M., Cortes, Y. I., & Caceres, B. A. (2021). Comparative effectiveness of behavioral interventions for cardiovascular risk reduction in Latinos: A systematic review. *Journal of Cardiovascular Nursing*. Advance online publication. https://doi.org/10.1097/JCN.0000000000000806

National Academies of Sciences, Engineering, and Medicine. (2021). *The future of nursing 2020–2030: Charting a path to achieve health equity*. National Academies Press. https://doi.org/10.17226/25982

National Advisory Council on Nurse Education and Practice. (2020). *Integration of social determinants of health in nursing education, practice, and research*. US Department of Health and Human Services. https://www.hrsa.gov/sites/default/files/hrsa/advisory-committees/nursing/reports/nacnep-2019-sixteenthreport.pdf

Russo, R. G., Li, Y., Đoàn, L. N., Ali, S. H., Siscovick, D., Kwon, S. C., & Yi, S. S. (2021). COVID-19, social determinants of health, and opportunities for preventing cardiovascular disease: A conceptual framework. *Journal of the American Heart Association*, *10*(24), e022721. https://doi.org/10.1161/JAHA.121.022721

White, B. M., Rochell, J. K., & Warren, J. R. (2020). Promoting cardiovascular health for African American women: An integrative review of interventions. *Journal of Women's Health*, *29*(7), 952–970. https://doi.org/10.1089/jwh.2018.7580

Zhang, Y., Zhang, Y., Sholle, E., Abedian, S., Sharko, M., Turchioe, M. R., Wu, Y., & Ancker, J. S. (2020). Assessing the impact of social determinants of health on predictive models for potentially avoidable 30-day readmission or death. *PLoS ONE*, *15*(6), e0235064. https://doi.org/10.1371/journal.pone.0235064

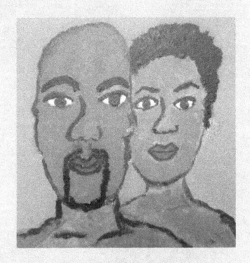

DREAMER

Last night I became a dreamer
I was lost in my thoughts of endless possibilities
What will tomorrow bring?
Who will I be when I emerge from this continuous fight?
Just to exist in peace
I dreamed of a space where I had the courage to be my authentic Black self
Where I could live without boundaries
Live without fear
Where I could shine without the trauma of battle wounds,
Without enemies in my path that will try to defeat me over and over again
I dreamed of a place where everyone could see
My beautiful shade of Blackness and
Understand the history my color represents
The beauty of my humanity
I dream of a painless existence
I dream of happiness
I dream of opportunities
I dream of freedom
Last night, I became a dreamer

Poetry and artwork by Lucinda Canty, PhD, CNM, FACNM
Associate Professor of Nursing, University of Massachusetts Amherst

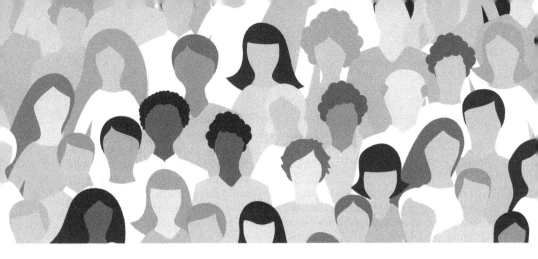

5 Multi-Sector Collaboration

In This Chapter

Nurses work in many areas within and outside of healthcare, and this chapter addresses some of those multi-sector collaborations. We are passionate about our duties regarding those we support and serve and often personally take full responsibility for outcomes. Although this is noble, we must recognize that we cannot be everything to everyone, and some challenges require help from those who possess other talents. We are experts at interprofessional collaboration within the context of healthcare, but people's lives extend far beyond the traditional healthcare setting. Acknowledging the contributions of those outside of healthcare and initiating, cultivating, and sustaining those collaborative relationships is imperative for successfully attaining health equity and building a cultural of health.

Consider the following questions as you read the essays about health equity and multi-sector collaboration:

- In what ways can nurses collaborate with other sectors to promote health equity?

- What are some examples of unlikely collaborations between nurses and other professions that have proven successful?

- List steps to cultivating a diverse coalition of partners to support health equity efforts.

- What nursing-specific challenges might benefit from multi-sector collaborations?

- What non-nursing professions have the potential to advance health equity?

The Unexpected Power (and Joy) of Cross-Sector Collaborations

Linda A. McCauley, PhD, RN, FAAN, FAAOHN
Dean and Professor, Emory University Nell Hodgson Woodruff School of Nursing

Inever knew what I wanted to be—as a first-generation college student, I was not even aware of how to be a college student. I quickly felt that I was an imposter in the college environment, where I believed the only thing of value I had to offer was my love for studying and learning. In high school, my role model was my mother, who was a diploma-educated nurse, and I learned to love work from her—an attribute that many nurses hold and that has influenced me for more than five decades. I followed in her path and began to work in the hospital at an early age, an experience that underscored for me the importance of respecting all people, regardless of race, age, education, or other factors. This early professional experience was invaluable, but I had limited options as a teenager: Women were expected to be nurses, secretaries, or teachers. No one ever talked to me about how to prepare for graduate school. Though I knew I loved medicine and healthcare, no one explained to me the many possible career paths in healthcare. I would sit for hours and study my mother's old anatomy and physiology textbooks from nursing school. I loved chemistry and mentioned to my mother one day that I thought being a pharmacist would be an interesting career. Her response was, "Why would you want to count pills all day?" And that was the end of that. Next, I thought I would love to be a physician; but coming from a family that barely "got by," I assumed I was too poor to follow that path. As a freshman taking mandatory classes in foreign languages, my professor asked me how he could help me study in France and major in that discipline. I was stunned. My calculus professor commented that I was gifted in math, but I had no clue what one did with a math degree except to become a schoolteacher. Isn't that sad? What I am trying to say is that first-generation students often have traveled a very narrow path to get to college. They have a passion, they've built on dreams, but many barriers can keep them from seeing possibilities and envisioning an overall journey.

Some first-generation students are fortunate to develop a relationship with a mentor during their college years. That did not happen to me. I remember my math, French, and chemistry professors, but not a single nursing professor had a significant impact on my journey. Not a single nursing faculty knew what I was struggling with as a first-generation student. I graduated from nursing thinking I had missed something larger than nursing. Today I have discovered that larger world of interdisciplinary, cross-sector work. I never lost my passion for math—I revisited it with a doctorate in epidemiology. I never lost my passion for chemistry—I revisited it in my research programs, in the science of environmental health, toxicology, and the impact of exposures on human health. I even revisited my passion for foreign languages, working for decades with vulnerable populations that do not speak English. But what I learned from my journey is how much I thrive when I have opportunities to work broadly and with a reach far beyond nursing. There is joy is studying how others approach problems in healthcare, and I am convinced that cross-disciplinary or cross-sector collaborations are essential in solving the complex issues of health inequity in our country and globally.

Nursing cannot improve health and reduce inequities alone. I remember my first large research grant for studying pesticide exposures among children of immigrant farmworkers. I had assembled a team of community health workers, neurologists, toxicologists, and social scientists, all working together in the paradigm of community-based participatory research. Perhaps speaking from a narrow perspective of nursing, a social epidemiologist said to me, what is your role on this team? I laughingly replied, my role was to bring this wild, crazy group together! But seriously, I realized for the first time that my broad interest in other fields, my education as a nurse who loves community health, and my desire to work with and support marginalized populations had come together in a beautiful way. I continue today, with my research and leadership roles, to believe that we are best when we collaborate with others and bring diverse opinions and points of view to the table. As Mother Teresa said, "None of us, including me, ever does great things. But we can all do small things, with great love, and together we can do something wonderful."

"Knowing there are such exceptional nurse leaders like Dr. Hassmiller around the world who dedicate their lives to improving the human condition is humbling and makes me want to be a better nurse. Multi-sector collaboration is the essence of our practice, steeped in a long tradition of caring for those in need, with a keen eye for health equity and the eradication of racism, sexism, ageism, and all the ways we as a society diminish those around us. Read this with the optimism that we can and will accomplish the changes we want to see."

–Terry Fulmer, PhD, RN, FAAN
President, the John A. Hartford Foundation

Going Together

Tay Kopanos, DNP, FNP, FAANP
Vice President of State Government Affairs,
American Association of Nurse Practitioners

In 2007, I had the opportunity to work on a legislative campaign with the Colorado Nurses Association. The goal was to address healthcare disparities and delays in care that result when the signatures of advanced practice registered nurses (APRN) are not accepted on various state forms related to patient care: forms for items like handicap parking license plates, verification of pregnancy for Medicaid eligibility, and certification of serious health conditions to prevent utility/power disconnection. It was a campaign that we all believed in, and the issue was straightforward: Nurses were already authorized to treat the patients but not their paperwork. That disconnect created delays, missed opportunities for care, and unnecessary costs by requiring a patient to see two healthcare providers to have one form signed.

"As a nurse focused on policy and implementing change, I'm very aware of the importance of reaching beyond nursing to accomplish our big goals. And as we face our preeminent national challenge today of achieving health equity built on strengthened nursing capacity and expertise, we as nurse leaders should be the bridges to other sectors that will help us accomplish this goal. We need allies in business, government, and academia; in social justice and consumer organizations; and in the other health professions—all of whom understand the valuable role that nurses play and can weave nursing through all aspects of our communities and institutions."

—Susan Reinhard, PhD, RN, FAAN
Senior Vice President and Director,
AARP Public Policy Institute
Chief Strategist, Center to Champion Nursing in America and
Family Caregiving Initiatives

Armed with the facts, figures, and a belief that legislators would see the issue as we did, we headed into legislative hearings. The bill failed to progress. In truth, it bombed. The issue that had been was so crystal clear to us wasn't tangible to legislators. "It can't be that hard to find someone else to sign these forms," commented a legislator. "I'm not sure the frequency of this is significant enough to warrant changing the law," added another. We had underestimated the knowledge that legislators had around the preparation of APRNs and the services they were providing patients. "I'm not sure that nurses should be providing this type of care. Is it safe?" asked legislators. Instead of discussing forms and paperwork, we found ourselves reviewing the rigor of graduate nursing education and defending clinical practice laws. We were also unprepared to counter the work that the state medical society had done in advance of the hearing to raise concerns about the bill. "The holes in this bill are big enough that you could drive a Mack truck through it," was one of the last comments made before the committee voted to defeat the legislation.

It was painful and frustrating. It would be a year before we could bring a bill back and try again. Another year of delays in care, missed opportunities, and unnecessary costs.

As we began to regroup, we knew that facts alone would not be enough. Our team sought out and met with organizations who had an overlapping interest in the same patient populations APRNs were treating. We highlighted how the lack of signature recognition impacted their business or individuals they represented. We successfully recruited many of these organizations to be part of the coalition, lend their lobbying support, and tell legislators about the challenges that they encountered when an outdated law prevented APRNs from handling the patient's paperwork. In the months leading up to the session we enlisted nurses and other healthcare providers from across the state to be part of the grassroots effort. We trained them how to connect with legislators and then called on them to engage before the hearing.

On the day of the hearing the following year, those opposing the legislation testified first. For more than half an hour individuals opposed to the legislation shared their opinion that signing these forms was not the practice of nursing and that it would be unsafe to allow APRNs to sign these forms for patients. When the opponents concluded, proponents of the bill were invited to testify. I was the first speaker. As I began to say my name and share that I was testifying in support of the bill on behalf of the Colorado Nurses Association, the chair of the committee stood up and began walking around the hearing room whispering with each committee member. Within a minute, the committee chair sat back down and interrupted my testimony. "Ms. Kopanos," he began, "it's clear that you and your colleagues are passionate about this issue. I've just polled my fellow committee members, and with your permission we'd like to vote. There are several other items on our docket that we want to get to, and we're ready to move on." I sat stunned. "Not again. You need to hear why this is so important," I thought. At that moment, the lobbyist for the Colorado Nurses Association who was sitting behind me nudged my chair and whispered, "Tay, let them vote." Reluctantly, I agreed and found myself saying, "Thank you, Mr. Chairman. Please vote."

As a roll-call vote was called, one-by-one each committee member voted in favor of the legislation. The bill unanimously passed the committee without the need to hear a word of supporting testimony! That was incredible. The bill continued to gain support throughout the rest of the legislative process, and two months later, it was signed into law by Governor Ritter.

The success of this legislation was the result of multiple partners working together to show the impact of outdated laws on patients and supporting a specific solution. Having worked on hundreds of pieces of legislation since, the lesson of that hearing remains fresh: If we are going to go, we must go together.

Here's how to begin to cultivate a diverse coalition of partners for health equity efforts:

- Look for partners who share overlapping patient populations, values, or vision.

- Clearly articulate what the issue is, how it impacts them/what they care about, why the proposed solution is the one to support, and why they should spend resources to support it now.

- Engage and include healthcare providers from outside of nursing.

- Integrate partners who can speak about the business impact, like employers and payers.

- Ensure balance by recruiting partners from all sides of the political spectrum.

- Be a partner—look for opportunities to lend your voice and influence support for efforts other associations are running.

Commitment to Advancing Health Equity With Hispanic/Latinx Communities Through Multi-Sector Collaboration

Adriana Perez, PhD, CRNP, ANP-BC, FAAN, FGSA
Associate Professor of Nursing
Senior Fellow, Leonard Davis Institute of Health Economics
University of Pennsylvania School of Nursing

One of the most important competencies of our nursing core education at the University of Pennsylvania School of Nursing is collaboration with others to make health a human right, to make healthcare accessible and equitable for marginalized communities, and to speak up against systems/policies perpetuating racism, ableism, ageism, sexism, and other forms of oppression. The latter is easier said than done; however, through collaboration, we develop courage knowing we are not alone in creating a better present and future. Multi-sector collaboration involves reaching out beyond the healthcare sector because health is shaped by multifactorial experiences related to education, housing, income, immigration status, and indigeneity, among many other factors. The complexity of these issues and historical trauma embedded in long-standing health inequities calls for different perspectives and comprehensive solutions that not one single sector can answer alone. This is good news. We do not have to know all the answers.

Key to collaboration is meaningful inclusion of persons/communities we aim to serve, and the challenge of inequities is indeed an important concern for the community. Our humility and willingness to learn from others, sharing our own knowledge, time, and commitment to do hard work can foster successful collaborations. There are challenges along the way, and rewards can come from celebrating small steps forward.

Tiempo Juntos por Nuestra Salud—which means "time together for our health"—is a multi-level physical activity intervention for older Latinos with mild cognitive impairment, developed through community collaborations. It was inspired by Hispanic/Latino elders in North Philadelphia, which also became the subject of my research. For six years, I immersed myself in the community as a nurse practitioner and researcher providing primary care services. I also served as an active collaborator, joining the Latino Golden Age Coalition of local Latino leaders with a mission to promote health and wellness for residents through the golden age years.

Tiempo Juntos is funded by the National Institutes of Health/National Institute on Aging, currently in its first year of implementation in partnership with organizations that contributed to the grant application (shared data to conceptualize the problem, described the local setting/population, and informed the recruitment plan and design of the physical activity intervention). In this example, when starting neighborhood group walks, the community adopted a Spanish *dicho* [saying], *"poco a poco, juntos llegamos lejos,"* or "little by little, together we can go far," which reaffirms the participants are doing their best.

As I learned, one of the first steps involving multi-sector collaboration was connecting with those already doing this work. Members of the coalition represent faith-based organizations, non-profits, social workers, legal services, and advocates with a 25-year history of serving the community. When purpose and mission align, collaboration comes easier. Despite all I read in the literature regarding being "hard to reach" and "lack of Latino participation in clinical trials," I saw a community interested in being active in research to bring needed resources and opportunities to address their priority health concerns: memory health and sleep.

An important next step in this multi-sector collaboration was ensuring that health priorities and concerns were defined from the perspective of the community of focus, in this case Spanish-speaking elders with memory problems and their family or care partners. Similarly, solutions had to reflect their values, concerns, and recommendations. Coalition stakeholders supported organizing focus groups at senior centers and health centers known to provide bilingual services. Being a bilingual/bicultural nurse scientist made a difference for me; however, partnering with local native speakers ensured an understanding of subcultural nuances and language differences.

Key findings included:

- Older Hispanics/Latinos want to preserve their treasured memories, serving as health role models for younger generations.

- Any program/intervention has to be offered in groups, as learning and remembering is better when done together.

- Flexibility in scheduling is important to most, who often have multiple healthcare and specialty appointments and family/church activities, or who might have to travel back home to their country of origin.

Meaningful collaboration takes time and commitment. An ongoing step of *Tiempo Juntos* includes formal involvement of community advisory board members who are compensated for their expertise in order to provide a platform for continued collaboration. They share unique expertise in marketing, communication, human resources, leadership development, and services dealing with nutrition, transportation, and spirituality. We all worked towards broader community/neighborhood level goals. Through the COVID-19 pandemic, I joined local leaders in connecting senior residents to Spanish resources and trusted information on COVID-19. Many asked me to share what I was seeing from a clinical perspective and nationally as guidelines evolved. We became trusted colleagues/friends bringing packaged food and care kits to Spanish-speaking seniors who were isolated and lonely.

Even the best of collaborations experience challenges; however, many of our challenges arose from logistical issues, differing views on reaching goals, or lack of clarity regarding expectations. Table 5.1 includes our common challenges and strategies we formulated to move forward.

Table 5.1. Multi-Sector Collaboration Challenges With Potential Strategies to Resolve

Challenges	Potential Strategies
Meeting/activity conflict in scheduling	Commit to being present and ready to contribute.
	If you miss anything, stay updated on outcomes, next steps, and ways you can still assist.
	Ask if you can join remotely; since COVID-19, time and space are not a major issue.
Differing views	Take time to listen intently. You can learn and grow from letting others lead.
	Learn the history.
	Share your experience and ideas.
	Set ego aside to remain focused on the goal.
Unclear expectations	It is good to ask questions.
	Share any limitations you may have openly.
	Work in good faith to resolve any conflict early on.

A key recommendation of this research was the inclusion and employment of community health promoters (CHPs), resident leaders who had graduated from a local CHP training program to lead walking groups and assist with sustainability. Multi-sector collaboration now includes working with national partners/stakeholders to address systemic barriers that exclude Hispanics/Latinos and other non-English speakers from participating in research, ensuring access to equitable healthcare and early detection/memory screenings, and economic relief for care partners through national paid family leave policies.

Little by little, together we WILL go far!

The School Nurses' Collaborative Role in Health Equity for Students

Donna Mazyck, MS, RN, LCPC, NCSN, NCC, CAE, FNASN
Executive Director, National Association of School Nurses

Advancing population health and health equity requires multi-sector collaboration among individuals, communities, and organizations/agencies, and no one knows this better than school nurses.

As a school nurse consultant in a state education agency, I heard from school health services leaders in school districts that gaps existed in vision screening education for health services staff. Vision and eye health facilitated learning for students. Inequities existed where students were unable to access vision exams and vision aids (e.g., eyeglasses or contact lenses). To address the health services staff education, I collaborated with two state vision care professional associations to travel across regions in the state to conduct training. In addition, we invited public health professionals to join the collaboration. To round out the vision and eye health collaborative, we advocated for evidence-based school vision screening cadence for preK-12 students in the state legislature. In some locations, community partners collaborated with schools to provide for students' vision exams and corrective lenses at the schools. This multi-sector collaboration addressed social needs for students and their families.

School nurses know students and their families over generations, giving an opportunity to observe, learn, and assess the social determinants of health that factor into family health and well-being (Schroeder et al., 2018). For example, school nurses link families and students with community-based services that provide food, vision care services, and transportation to appointments. Such collaborations on local levels flow from community connections and relationships built over time. Collaboration enables discovery of social determinants of health, social influencers of health and education, and social needs that adversely affect individual and population-based health and well-being. Nurses, especially in community settings, have collaborated with organizations, agencies, and individuals to address individual social needs with clients.

Nurses do whole-person assessments that allow discovering and providing for client social needs, most often with knowledge of resources in healthcare systems or in community agencies. Nurses ask, what is the presenting concern? What worries them? How did they travel to the appointment? Nurses follow a process that begins with assessment, which involves critical thinking, observation, and data collection. Those skills and the ability to make a nursing diagnosis, perform client-centered planning, implement the plan, and evaluate the results are skills nurses offer in multi-sector collaborations. Access to low or no cost transportation, healthy and safe housing, and affordable and nutritious food can result in desirable outcomes for client health. Simply put, these midstream solutions for social needs are helpful on an individual level.

However, systems-level upstream changes drive the predominant improvement of health inequities. Improved health inequities result from addressing community conditions through policy change and multi-sector collaboration (Castrucci & Auerbach, 2019). Multi-sector collaboration including nurses and other disciplines, healthcare systems, public health entities, community organizations, and social sectors contain the components necessary to address complexities that social factors cause in under-resourced communities (National Academies of Sciences, Engineering, and Medicine, 2021). Nurses bring wholistic client/patient perspectives to multi-sector collaborations, and with strong advocacy skills, they can have significant effects on upstream changes.

Multi-sector collaborations require intentional actions to form and maintain focus on a shared agenda. With work across sectors—whether federal, state, or regional; whether public or private—challenges exist in tackling population-based social determinants of health. Healthcare, public health, and social sectors move the needle on systems change related to social determinants of health when they align across four areas (Lanford et al., 2021):

1. Developing a shared purpose with the community at stake, both formally and informally

2. Clearly defining roles. Roles include leadership in individual and collaborative sectors. A backbone organization can convene the collaboration; community involvement enriches the collaborative.

3. Finding funding and managing resources

4. Sharing data

Example: A successful multi-sector collaboration formed to address families who experienced social and economic factors that adversely affected client health and well-being. The partnership included a nurse family partnership program and other healthcare providers and support services. Nurses who made home visits to pregnant and parenting women formed trusted, respectful, and valued relationships with clients. Williams et al. (2021) listed contributing elements for this effective collaboration:

- Relational in nature, with committed leadership and provider champions

- Shared perceptions of trust, respect, and value

- Mission similarity between providers

- Integrated policies and systems (e.g., data sharing and communication channels)

Riley et al. (2021) found that a framework for systems that successfully collaborate achieve goals when aligned in four areas: the problems, the mechanisms, the solutions, and goal attainment.

Multi-sector collaborations hold promise for improving population health and advancing health equity. Research can shed light on what helps multi-sector collaborations accomplish structural systems change that address social determinants of health. To advance health equity for populations, nurses, especially school nurses, thrive in multi-sector collaboratives.

References

Castrucci, B. C., & Auerbach, J. (2019, January 16). Meeting individual social needs falls short of addressing social determinants of health. *HealthAffairs*. https://www.healthaffairs.org/do/10.1377/hblog20190115.234942

Lanford, D., Petiwala, A., Landers, G., & Minyard, K. (2021). Aligning healthcare, public health and social services: A scoping review of the role of purpose, governance, finance, and data. *Health & Social Care in the Community, 30*(1), 432–447. https://doi.org/10.1111/hsc.13374

National Academies of Sciences, Engineering, and Medicine. (2021). *The future of nursing 2020–2030: Charting a path to achieve health equity.* National Academies Press. https://www.ncbi.nlm.nih.gov/books/NBK573898/

Riley, W. J., Love, K., Runger, G., Shafer, M., Pine, K., & Mays, G. (2021). Framework for multi-sector alignment research. *Journal of Public Health Management and Practice, 27*(5), E205–E209. doi:10.1097/PHH.0000000000001275

Schroeder, K., Malone, S. K., McCabe, E., & Lipman, T. (2018). Addressing the social determinants of health: A call to action for school nurses. *The Journal of School Nursing, 34*(3), 182–191. https://doi.org/10.1177/1059840517750733

Williams, V. N. G., McManus, B. M., Brooks-Russell, A., Yost, E., Allison, M. A., Olds, D. L., & Tung, G. J. (2021). A qualitative study of effective collaboration among nurse home visitors, healthcare providers, and community support services in the United States. *Health & Social Care in the Community, 30*(5), 1881–1893. https://doi.org/10.1111/hsc.13567

Taking Advantage of a Crisis to Forge New Multi-Sector Collaborations

Garrett K. Chan, PhD, APRN, FAEN, FPCN, FNAP, FCNS, FAANP, FAAN
President & CEO, HealthImpact

In March of 2020, the United States implemented isolation mandates for most people living and working in communities in an effort to slow the SARS-CoV-2 virus infection and death rates. However, during the pandemic, not all members of society could stay home. Essential workers played an important role in ensuring that communities could continue to have access to healthcare, environmental services, groceries, and household essential goods. These essential workers were largely from communities of color and at a higher risk of contracting COVID-19.

HealthImpact, a 501(c)3 nonprofit organization, is the California nursing workforce and policy center. In late 2020, HealthImpact realized there would be three "bottlenecks" or challenges to reaching herd immunity. The first bottleneck would be the lack of vaccine supply and the number of doses available for vaccination. As the vaccine supply increased, the second bottleneck would be the lack of healthcare workers available to administer the vaccine and the lack of venues for the public to access the vaccine, especially in under-resourced communities and communities of color. The third bottleneck would be the public perspective of vaccine hesitancy. As a result of the bottleneck analysis, HealthImpact created VaxForce—a California-wide volunteer workforce management system to vet healthcare professionals and students and match them with existing vaccination events or create VaxForce-led vaccination events in partnership with local community-based organizations (CBOs) and county public health departments.

VaxForce was created using the HandsOn Connect (2022) volunteer management platform. HandsOn Connect was instrumental in supporting the creation of VaxForce because of its focus on health equity, and the staff worked hard to get VaxForce established for quick deployment of the system. VaxForce played two critical roles. First, it served as a volunteer recruitment and deployment system to manage the volunteer workforce by conducting background checks, verifying competencies, and delineating the California regions in which the volunteers would work. Second, VaxForce coordinated community vaccination events and posted them within the system for the volunteers to match themselves with which vaccination events they wanted to work.

VaxForce collaborated with local CBOs in underserved regions of California to support vaccination events in their communities, especially in communities that had barriers of distance, time, and lack of access to vaccinations. Partnering with CBOs is imperative, as they have already established trust in their communities and are essential in any effort to increase health equity given that trust and acquired knowledge of the needs, correct approaches, and established relationships with informal community leaders. VaxForce also worked with county public health departments and other healthcare agencies to procure the needed vaccines. Each collaborating agency had very important roles and responsibilities in creating this type of collaboration.

A series of vaccine events were held in a farmland community in rural Sacramento County. Rachel Rios, CEO, and Mao Vang, Youth and Health Program Manager of La Familia Counseling Center in Sacramento, approached HealthImpact because they wanted to provide vaccines to farmworkers who had no local access to vaccines or healthcare. To offer these events, the leadership team needed to work with other CBOs. Table 5.2 delineates which organizations were primarily responsible and their roles and responsibilities:

Table 5.2 Community-Based Organizational Roles in Vaccine Deployment

Roles & Responsibilities	Organizations
Procuring the interprofessional licensed vaccination staff and students	HealthImpact and VaxForce
	Sigma Zeta Eta at-Large Chapter
	American Nurses Association/California
	Association of California Nurse Leaders
Procuring the lay volunteers for the event	La Familia Counseling Center
	Latino Economic Council of Sacramento
	Angels in the Field
	Casa de Español
	Direct Relief
	First 5 Sacramento
	California Human Development Corporation
Procuring the vaccine	Sacramento Native American Health Center
	Sacramento Department of Public Health
Determining the location and setting up the vaccine event	La Familia Counseling Center
	Sacramento Farm Bureau
	Kay Dix Farms

continues

Table 5.2 Community-Based Organizational Roles in Vaccine Deployment   (cont.)

Roles & Responsibilities	Organizations
Registering the vaccine recipients	La Familia Counseling Center
	Kay Dix Farms
Publicizing the event	La Familia Counseling Center
	Lilly Cortes Wyatt Public Relations
	Kay Dix Farms
	Latino Economic Council of Sacramento
	Angels in the Field
	Casa de Español
Enhancing vaccine confidence in the community to sign up vaccine recipients	La Familia Counseling Center
	Angels in the Field
	Casa de Español
	Direct Relief
	First 5 Sacramento
	California Human Development Corporation

Through this partnership and series of events, we learned several valuable lessons including the importance of establishing clear roles and responsibilities for each step of the process, understanding the local logistics and unique issues within the community, and identifying additional CBO partners that already had existing relationships in the community. Working with organizations that are courageous and nimble enough to create novel innovations and who prioritize the goal of health equity above previous policies and procedures that constrain rather than free up creative thinking is essential in transforming services to improve health equity. As a result of these lessons learned, the team was able to create subsequent successful events that were interprofessional, demonstrated successes of outcomes and working together, created more opportunities in new areas, garnered more trust within the community, and achieved health equity outcomes.

Since March 2021, VaxForce has mobilized 315 health professional volunteers in 71 vaccination events, administering over 8,200 vaccines. VaxForce established relationships with over 20 CBOs. The racial and ethnic profile of vaccine recipients in VaxForce events is 48% Latinx, 25% Black, 4% Asian, 20% white, and 3% mixed race. All VaxForce events have been held in communities designated by the Centers for Disease Control and Prevention (CDC) as moderate to severe for COVID-19 vulnerability, and 86% of VaxForce events have been held in communities designated as moderate vulnerability and high vulnerability by the CDC's Social Vulnerability Index (Agency for Toxic Substance & Disease Registry, 2020). Additionally, 59% of VaxForce events have been held in areas designated by the CDC as hesitant and hesitant or unsure about COVID-19 vaccines.

References

Agency for Toxic Substance & Disease Registry (2020). *CDC/ATSDR Social Vulnerability Index*. https://www.atsdr.cdc.gov/placeandhealth/svi/index.html

HandsOn Connect Cloud Solutions. (2022). *Home*. https://www.handsonconnect.com/

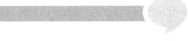

Addressing Health Equity Together

Lauran Hardin, MSN, RN-BC, CNL, FNAP
Vice President & Senior Advisor, National Healthcare & Housing Advisors, LLC

Solving complex problems can seem insurmountable: homelessness, substance use disorder, food insecurity, domestic violence, a laundry list of challenges underscored by poverty and trauma. As a nurse I have spent more than two decades caring for the most complex populations. I learned that addressing deep-rooted systemic problems is not something we do alone. The core competencies of our profession have positioned nurses to lead in addressing health equity and to do so through powerful collaborations.

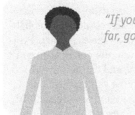

"If you want to go fast, go alone; but if you want to go far, go together."

–African Proverb

Learn From Individuals

My best teacher was a young man who had more than 50 emergency room visits in three different hospital systems across the city in one year. Individually, our health systems provided evidence-based care for what was presented in the moment, but none of us were addressing the root cause of what was really happening. He continued to cycle through the revolving door of our systems until we took a different approach.

Like many others who frequently access the healthcare system, he had needs that we weren't assessing or listening to: He was homeless, hungry, and lonely. Until we integrated comprehensive assessment, including screening for his health-related social needs, we were missing the real reason he was returning to the health system. Integrating social determinants of health screening is a core practice all nurses can adapt to start the foundation for addressing health equity.

Understanding his story led us to think differently about delivery of care. The team that was caring for him extended far outside the hospital walls including homeless services, community agencies, behavioral health providers, the police, and EMS providers. We convened a case conference across sectors to develop a shared plan of care integrating providers across sectors into one cross continuum team to address his needs (Vest et al., 2018). Coordination led to consistency in his care, integration of behavioral health at the point of care, a coordinated approach to housing, and resolution of long unmet needs. Case conferencing is emerging as a best practice in addressing coordination of care and is being integrated in payment structures such as the enhanced care management benefit in the redesign of Medicaid in California (State of California Health and Human Services Agency, Department of Healthcare Services, 2021). Regardless of setting, nurses can initiate this kind of collaborative approach to comprehensively meet health equity needs.

Act as a Community

Learning from individuals quickly takes us to seeing the opportunity to address another level of need. Communities are coming together across sectors to collaboratively build collective responses to address health equity. One example is Project Restoration in Lake County, California, where a community collaborative of healthcare, social services, behavioral health, police, EMS, and community-based organizations work together to serve the needs of their most vulnerable community members (Hardin et al., 2020). Sharing data across sectors, they identify people with the most frequent access to their systems and reach out together to address needs. Lessons learned from individual intervention are shared, and the community works together to build the resources to address root causes.

Over a five-year period, the community built a resource navigation center, services for the homeless, transitional housing, access to behavioral health, access to substance use treatment, and collaborative pathways to connect agencies in an efficient delivery system to address health equity. People served in the program are connected to a pathway to share their lived experience with others through mentorship and job opportunities. Together they have created a stronger community ecosystem for marginalized populations that has generated greater than 40% reduction in unnecessary system utilization and cost and created improved health outcomes, access to benefits, food security, and housing. Nurses are well positioned to lead and contribute to these types of emerging collaboratives.

Create Systems-Level Change

Deeply impacting health equity requires collaboration at the highest level to change structural root causes affecting populations. More than 60 healthcare systems across the country have joined forces in the Healthcare Anchor Network to collectively leverage assets to catalyze community collaboration (2022). Their focus is to address the root causes of economic and racial inequities that negatively impact individual, family, and community health and well-being. Initiatives include place-based investments, building affordable housing, and addressing workforce issues.

Creating structures for competitors to collaborate is key to advancing these types of initiatives. Nurse leaders can start by initiating a collective approach within their own organizations to look at process improvement opportunities to address health-related social needs like access to benefits or food security (Hardin et al., 2017). Taking that approach to community partners will extend the impact by working together across community systems to address root causes. If the leadership role extends beyond the local community, consider how the organization can use its circle of influence to bring together cross-sector actors into collaborative action around a shared need. For example, the Community Benefit Collaborative is a collective of system-level community benefit leaders from Kaiser, CommonSpirit, Trinity Health, Adventist Health, and Providence Saint Joseph health systems. Their footprint covers more than 30 states, and they are sharing resources to collectively address social needs like investing together to end chronic homelessness in a healthcare and homeless system integration pilot (Community Solutions, n.d.).

Together We Can

Regardless of our role or position, we have an opportunity to build a shared table to address health equity. Clients and communities are asking for a different approach. Alone there is only so much we can accomplish. Together we can do so much more. Our collective action will take us across the finish line to sustainable change.

References

Community Solutions. (n.d.). *Health care and homelessness*. https://community.solutions/health-care-and-homelessness

Hardin, L., Kilian, A., & Spykerman, K. (2017). Competing health systems and complex patients: An interprofessional collaboration to improve outcomes and reduce healthcare costs. *Journal of Interprofessional Education and Practice, 7*(6), 5–10. https://doi.org/10.1016/j.xjep.2017.01.002

Hardin, L., Trumbo, S. & Wiest, D. (2020). Cross-sector collaboration for vulnerable populations reduces utilization and strengthens community partnerships. *Journal of Interprofessional Education and Practice, 18*(3), 5–10. https://doi.org/10.1016/j.xjep.2019.100291

Healthcare Anchor Network. (2022). *About the Healthcare Anchor Network*. https://healthcareanchor.network/about-the-healthcare-anchor-network/

National Academies of Sciences, Engineering and Medicine. (2019). *Integrating social care into the delivery of health care: Moving upstream to improve the nation's health.* The National Academies Press. https://doi.org/10.17226/25467

State of California Health and Human Services Agency, Department of Health Care Services. (2021). CalAIM Enhanced care management policy guide. https://www.dhcs.ca.gov/Documents/MCQMD/ECM-Policy-Guide-September-2021.pdf

Vest, J., Caine, V., Harris, L., Watson, D., Menachemi, N., & Halverson, P. (2018). Fostering local health department and health system collaboration through case conference for at-risk and vulnerable populations. *American Journal of Public Health, 108*(5), 649–651. https://doi.org/10.2105/AJPH.2018.304345

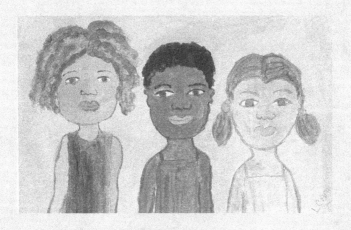

Rise Above

Unhealed wounds reopened
Exposing unexamined pain to the elements
The realization that my vulnerabilities are seen by
those who have the power to harm me.
Powerless in this system of oppression
Structures in place that leave me struggling to breathe

How do I find the courage to be my authentic self?
How do I find a place in a space that was not designed for me?
The answers were right in front of me
I went to my history and
Learned from my ancestors
I have a right to be here
A right to be heard
I found the strength to end this cycle of violence
I will rise above the structural barrier
Watch me, As I defy gravity

Poetry and artwork by Lucinda Canty, PhD, CNM, FACNM
Associate Professor of Nursing, University of Massachusetts Amherst

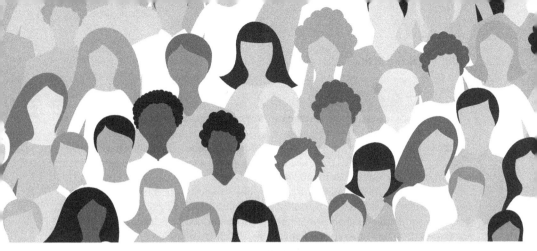

Preparing for Disasters and Public Health Emergencies

6

In This Chapter

- The American Red Cross: Volunteering in Times of Disasters

- Leveraging Disaster Recovery for Community Preparedness

- Disaster Response: Helping Those Who Help Others

- Preparing for Disasters and Public Health Emergencies

- Learning Lessons From COVID-19: Upstream Fishing to Mend Downstream Implications

This chapter considers how nursing can work to decrease the inequitable outcomes related to social determinants of health, structural racism, and environmental injustices that result from past and future disasters and public health emergencies. Nurses have used their keen assessment skills for centuries to support communities devastated by natural disasters. It is now time to elevate nursing education and continuing education to include substantive trainings focusing on disaster preparedness. As global warming continues to affect the quality and quantity of natural disasters, more nurses will need to be ready to provide care in non-clinical environments. Furthermore, the aid and care provided by these nurses will need to be guided by the competency and awareness of built environments that may perpetuate poor outcomes, and appropriate solutions will need to be created to foster health equity.

Consider the following questions as you read the essays about health equity and preparing for disasters and public health emergencies:

- How can nurses advocate for those who have experienced disasters and public health emergencies?

- With regards to being exposed to trauma, how can nurses protect their mental well-being?

- In what ways can nurses contribute to stabilizing communities that have experienced disasters and public health emergencies?

- What are characteristics of a community that may make its outcomes worse than others?

- How can the management of modern-day disasters and public health be guided by historical incidents that led to disparate outcomes?

The American Red Cross: Volunteering in Times of Disasters

Linda MacIntyre, PhD, RN, PHN, FAAN
Chief Nurse, American Red Cross

Nurses are the most trusted of professionals and have been named as a significant group that can achieve health equity by *The Future of Nursing* report (National Academies of Sciences, Engineering, and Medicine, 2021). Yet, *The Future of Nursing 2020–2030* report also states that many nurses are not prepared to address disasters and public health emergencies that disproportionally affect disadvantaged individuals.

The Environmental Protection Agency released a report stating that racial minorities in the US will bear a disproportionate burden of climate change effects, including more deaths from extreme heat and property loss from flooding in the wake of sea level rise (US Environmental Protection Agency, 2021). The Red Cross reports that "climate change impacts affect vulnerable populations" and that this increases the need for Red Cross services (2021).

Ninety percent of the American Red Cross workforce is comprised of volunteers. More volunteers, both those with a health professional license and those without a license, are needed to assist individuals and families to prepare for disasters, respond to disasters, and help individuals and communities recover from disasters.

> "As climate change, natural disasters, and emerging infectious disease outbreaks increasingly create hazards to human health, nurses' preparedness becomes ever more critical."
>
> –Tener Veenma, PhD
> Senior Scientist
> Department of International Health at the Johns Hopkins Bloomberg School of Public Health

As advocates, nurses must first ensure that they are personally prepared for disasters and emergencies. There are many resources to support well-being, and Dr. Kathryn Booth addresses resilience training later in this chapter ("Disaster Response: Helping Those Who Help Others"). Additionally, a disaster responder needs to complete a plan for all who depend upon them—for example, parents, children, neighbors, and pets. They also need a disaster kit, and finally, they need to take training to ensure that they have the confidence to respond.

Fortunately, training is available through the American Red Cross. The Red Cross provides extensive disaster training and uses an RN-led community nursing model for Disaster Health Services. In most US disasters, hospitals and emergency medical systems remain intact, but collaboration is key since assistance from neighboring areas may be needed. Responders should be prepared to provide basic first aid, for which the Red Cross offers classes and a free first aid mobile app. Individuals who need more extensive levels of care are generally referred to appropriate providers.

The Red Cross quickly organizes shelter and meals after a disaster. Nurses assess physical and mental/emotional status and the safety of the environment for individuals affected by disasters. Nurses consider social determinants of health—what needs does the individual/family have based on where they work, live, play, go to school, and worship? Are there factors that support or hinder their recovery based on social determinants of health? Are resources needed to address health equity?

Nurses assess medication and durable medical equipment needs. They listen carefully as individuals tell their stories and share their concerns. The Red Cross Disaster Health Services nurse helps a family with a child on the autism spectrum find a quiet place in a shelter and works with partners to ensure that headphones and weighted blankets are available as needed.

The Disaster Health Services team works closely with disaster mental health and advises individuals to avoid repeated exposure to media coverage of the disaster. Disaster Health Services nurses work with other health professionals to support disaster clients in maintaining independence. The nurse learns about resources to support individuals and families and communicates with other Red Cross teams and partners to ensure that disaster-related needs are met.

Just as a new nurse needs to understand the culture of their workplace—for example, how to use communication systems, obtain supplies, and work with other teams to ensure continuity of care—disaster responders learn about the disaster operation, chain of command, and how to obtain resources to ensure client needs are met. Disaster Health Services training initially takes about eight to nine hours, and nursing contact hours are available. For event-based volunteers who respond to a local disaster, there are often opportunities to support the disaster with minimal training. Ideally, a nurse will take necessary training before it is needed. This helps ensure they are prepared and will respond when needed.

I worked for the Red Cross in the Midwest and provided disaster training over several years for a faculty member's community health nursing course. One day, a nurse was needed for a shift in a shelter that was set up following a tornado. I asked the faculty member to take the shift, and she expressed concerns that she was unprepared. I explained that the primary role was to assess the disaster client needs and direct another nurse to assist where necessary. The Emergency Medical System was working, and if a disaster client needed assistance beyond what could be provided in the shelter, she was instructed to call 911. I also gave her my phone number should she have any questions. She agreed to take the shift, and the next day I thanked her profusely. The nurse stopped me and said, "No, thank *you*! I received so much more than I gave."

It is both humbling and an honor to be able to support someone after a disaster. I am acutely aware that I could be either the one assisting after a disaster or the one in need of assistance. Disaster needs may not arise for several days (Springer, 2013), and Red Cross disaster health and mental health workers ask individuals daily about their needs to support their disaster recovery. Nurses who consider the social determinants of health help identify both needs and resources to meet those needs.

Volunteers have found lifelong friends while supporting individual and community recovery from a disaster. As a Red Cross disaster volunteer, you can decide to respond locally or deploy to a disaster in another area. For deployed workers, all transportation, food, and lodging are provided by generous donors. I invite you to join the Red Cross health professional community and become a volunteer (https://www.redcross.org/volunteer/become-a-volunteer.html#). If you have questions, email us at RedCrossNurse@redcross.org. Together we can promote health equity for all.

References

American Red Cross. (2021). Red Cross statement on climate change. https://intranet. redcross.org/content/redcross/news/2021/09/update-on-our-climate-change-work.html

National Academies of Sciences, Engineering, and Medicine. (2021). *The future of nursing 2020–2030: Charting a path to achieve health equity.* National Academies Press. https:// nam.edu/publications/the-future-of-nursing-2020-2030

Springer, J. (2013). *Cot-to-cot: Identifying access and functional needs in community disaster shelters—What this means and how it applies to public health nursing practice.* https://www. maphn.org/Resources/Documents/Springer%20to%20Post%2007%2011%2013.pdf

US Environmental Protection Agency. (2021). *EPA report shows disproportionate impacts of climate change on socially vulnerable populations in the United States.* https://www.epa.gov/ newsreleases/epa-report-shows-disproportionate-impacts-climate-change-socially-vulnerable

Leveraging Disaster Recovery for Community Preparedness

Rear Admiral Aisha K. Mix, DNP, MPH, RN, NHDP-BC
Chief Nurse Officer, US Public Health Service

Disasters include incidents that jeopardize the health and safety of communities and the people within them. When a major disaster declaration has been made in the United States, there is a determination that the incident's severity is beyond the combined capabilities of the state and local governments to respond. The declaration acknowledges the gap between what is needed for the health and safety of the impacted communities and what the jurisdiction has the resources to address. The work that follows seeks to close the identified gaps to achieve maximum preparedness of the community and its members.

Reviewing the disaster cycle (see Figure 6.1), the most immediate period following the incident includes emergency management and response operations that are focused on stabilizing and sustaining essential community lifelines (Federal Emergency Management Agency, 2019). So, if we consider the response phase of a disaster or emergency as lifesaving, then the phase of recovery into prevention and mitigation can be considered life-sustaining. As we continue engaging through the cycle, the lessons learned during recovery begin to inform the community's next steps.

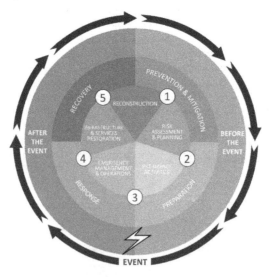

Figure 6.1 The disaster cycle.

An integral part of this process is reassessment of the community's needs, mitigation of identified risks, and design of a strategy that ensures the highest level of preparedness for future incidents. Understanding the health threats and risks that people experienced pre-disaster is important as we seek to predict or understand a community's or population's level of resilience following the incident. It is critical that this community assessment focus not only on the most marginalized people and the populations at highest risk for poor health outcomes, but also on identification of the community's strengths and opportunities to thrive. The whole community assessment, therefore, identifies pre-disaster deficits, assesses incident-related impacts, targets appropriate resources, and informs strategies to promote the health and well-being of individuals and communities.

Our ability to achieve and maintain health and well-being is impacted by many factors, including where we are born, live, learn, work, play, worship, and age (US Department of Health and Human Services, 2020). Referred to as *social determinants of health*, these factors can almost predict how well we navigate threats to health, especially during the response and recovery phases of a disaster. Consider these situations, as described by federal responders, that reflect social determinants and their impact on, or threat to, health:

- **Readiness for evacuation:** Age, level of ability, and preexisting health and social conditions became barriers to evacuation ahead of the disaster. Individuals chose not to evacuate because they were physically unable to or were caring for someone who was physically unable. Survivors of domestic violence had concerns about evacuating for fear that they would end up in the same shelter as their abuser.

- **Trust and/or fear:** Disenfranchised neighborhoods and communities, whether due to race, ethnicity, and/or economic status, expressed higher levels of mistrust and lower levels of interaction with the greater community. Until and unless a trusted member of the community presented the options, the community members were hesitant to listen and adhere to the instructions from responders.

The pre- and post-disaster assessments inform appropriate interventions that target one or more factors related to Healthy People 2030's Social Determinants of Health (Office of Disease Prevention and Health Promotion, n.d.) and trigger movement toward health equity:

- Healthcare access and quality

  - Assess: Resources and health-seeking behaviors of the community

  - Identify: Pre- and post-disaster barriers to obtaining quality health and behavioral health services

- Neighborhood and built environment

  - Assess: Infrastructure and supports for health and physical activity

  - Identify: Pre-disaster limitations and post-disaster exacerbation of existing needs for healthy community design

- Social and community context
  - Assess: Informal and formal leadership (e.g., gatekeepers) within the impacted populations and social factors, including political influence, racism, and roles of organizational networks
  - Identify: Social and human services capabilities and networks that promote independence of community members, especially children, seniors/elderly, and individuals with access and functional needs that impact their ability to access or receive care
- Economic stability
  - Assess: Critical, pre-disaster employment sectors and the contributions of the workforce
  - Identify: Post-disaster impacts for people who may no longer have steady work, have experienced injuries or conditions that limit their ability to work, or must change careers to achieve economic security
- Education access and quality
  - Assess: Resources for children and adolescents, including those with special healthcare needs and those not connected with the school system
  - Identify: Post-disaster impacts caused by closure of schools and/or reduction in resources and services usually provided

(US Department of Health & Social Services, 2020)

Health inequities occur when individuals or groups do not have the opportunity to attain their full health potential and, instead, are disadvantaged because of their social position or socially determined circumstances (Centers for Disease Control and Prevention, n.d.). While downstream or individual-level health services address immediate needs that occur during the response phase of a disaster, upstream initiatives must be identified and incorporated into the recovery phase to address the social and economic conditions that affect community health (Castrucci & Auerbach, 2019). Public health nurses are well-positioned to coordinate across sectors of the community, design programs and care delivery models that incorporate social determinants of health, and influence policy development to meet health and human service needs at the population levels (Castrucci & Auerbach, 2019).

Whether our nursing practice is in the acute, ambulatory care, or community setting, nurses collectively care for the whole person and the whole population. Disaster preparedness, which follows the recovery and mitigation phases, requires engagement from every one of us. Building upon our nursing foundation that focuses on protection, promotion, and optimization of health and abilities (American Nurses Association, 2021), the nurse's role in disaster preparedness is one that enhances community fortitude. While *resilience* describes an ability to bounce back or return to a prior state, *fortitude* describes the strength to encounter danger, pain, or adversity with courage (Merriam-Webster, 2022). Thus, community fortitude presents the true opportunity to incorporate pre-disaster strengths and position the community at its best when facing the next disaster or public health emergency.

References

American Nurses Association (2021). *Scope of practice.* https://nursingworld.org/practice-policy/scope-of-practice/

Castrucci, B., & Auerbach, J. (2019, January 16). Meeting individual social needs falls short of addressing social determinants of health. *HealthAffairs.* https://www.healthaffairs.org/do/10.1377/forefront.20190115.234942/full/

Centers for Disease Control and Prevention. (n.d.). *Health equity.* https://www.cdc.gov/chronicdisease/healthequity/index.htm

Federal Emergency Management Agency. (2019, October 28). *National response framework.* https://www.fema.gov/emergency-managers/national-preparedness/frameworks/response

Merriam-Webster. (2022). Fortitude. In *Merriam-Webster's dictionary.* https://www.merriam-webster.com/dictionary/fortitude

US Department of Health and Human Services, Office of Disease Prevention and Health Promotion. (n.d.). *Social determinants of health.* Healthy People 2030. https://health.gov/healthypeople/priority-areas/social-determinants-health

Disaster Response: Helping Those Who Help Others

Kathryn C. Booth, DNP, RN, CNL
Manager of Emergency Medical Services and Disaster Preparedness
Advocate Illinois Masonic Medical Center

If you've ever flown, you've most likely heard the instructions to put your oxygen mask on first before helping others. Why? Because you won't be able to help anyone if you run out of oxygen first. Why then do nurses and healthcare providers generally ignore this safety adage? We know that we can't help our patients if we don't first help ourselves, and yet we can't seem to help ourselves. So, how do we help the helpers responding to devastating disasters?

While most of the world paused at some point during the COVID-19 pandemic, weather-related events and natural disasters did not. Natural disasters have been increasing in severity for more than a decade (National Centers for Environmental Information, 2021). At the American Red Cross, this increased the demands for disaster response resources like volunteers, supplies, and deployment logistics. Red Cross disaster relief programs were acutely impacted by COVID-19 as the disaster season, more severe May through November, overlapped with the pandemic. Disaster response nurses supported individuals and families challenged with housing, transportation, food, and social isolation issues—social determinants that can lead to poor health and diminished well-being.

In the face of the persisting pandemic and increasingly severe disaster seasons, a program utilizing resilience-building techniques was implemented for Red Cross Nursing and Health Leaders (NHLs) in the late summer of 2021. The NHL group invited to pilot this program were 100 volunteer members across different US geographic regions who help manage disaster response, blood donation events, training services, and more, including frontline work and deployment.

> "Disasters, both natural and man-made, have turned from episodic to chronic due to climate change, infectious disease spread, and the unsettled social fabric of today's world. These events disproportionately affect individuals that are also affected by social determinants of health in a negative manner. Nurses are uniquely qualified to assist these individuals impacted by disaster due to their education to assist clients holistically. Therefore, it is paramount that nurses prepare, respond, and assist with recovery to disasters which will require education over and above current curricula. Now is the time to get ready to respond and act."
>
> —Mary Casey-Lockyer, MHS, BSN, RN, CCRN
> Disaster Health Services Program Lead,
> National Headquarters,
> American Red Cross

Working with NHLs from the height of COVID-19 in May 2020 through the summer of 2021, they expressed strong feelings of fatigue and burnout. They voiced being overwhelmed, disengaged, irritable, and even having trouble sleeping. Some attributed these stressors to the increased demands of disaster response programs and the overwhelming impact of COVID-19 on workforce, resources, and program delivery.

Literature shows that healthcare workers or first responders who witness suffering for prolonged periods of time are more likely to suffer from emotional exhaustion (Rushton et al., 2015). Such experiences are typical for NHLs who are deployed to disaster areas working the intake shelters, seeing neighborhoods destroyed, and helping families who have been devasted by wildfires or flooding. Work-related stressors and burnout, particularly in healthcare, can negatively impact mental health (Makwana, 2019; Rushton et al., 2015). Building resilience is an established technique to combat the effects of fatigue, stress, and burnout.

Try this for a few moments (HeartMath, 2021c):

- Focus your attention in the area of your heart. Imagine your breath is flowing in and out of your heart or chest area, breathing a little slower and deeper than usual. Suggestion: Inhale for five seconds and exhale for five seconds, or use whatever rhythm is comfortable.

- Make a sincere attempt to experience a regenerative feeling such as appreciation or care for someone or something in your life. Suggestion: Try to re-experience the feeling you have for someone you love—a pet, a special place, an accomplishment, etc.—or focus on a feeling of calm or ease.

What do you notice? Are you calmer? More focused on reading this? Or just wondering what this has to do with disaster nursing?

That was the HeartMath Quick Coherence technique.

HeartMath is a program that combines science-based techniques with coherence technology to empower people to self-regulate their emotions and behaviors with the goal of reducing stress, increasing resilience, and bringing balance (Heart-Math, 2021d). Different from meditation or deep-belly breathing, HeartMath is designed to be done in fast-paced environments for only a few moments to help focus attention and bring coherence between the heart rhythm and brain activity (HeartMath, 2021c). These techniques have been utilized on an organizational level at the Department of Veterans Affairs, Kaiser Permanente, and the National Aeronautics and Space Administration (HeartMath, 2021a).

HeartMath has demonstrated an average of 24% increase in focus, 30% increase in better sleep, and 38% increase in calmness (HeartMath, 2021b). A study specific to nursing found that over 400 nurses benefited from HeartMath with significant increases in goal clarity, work attitude, productivity, and communication effectiveness (Goldfisher et al., 2014).

A HeartMath workshop series was implemented at Red Cross to increase resilience for NHLs. This series was a voluntary six-week course of weekly one-hour sessions utilizing HeartMath resilience techniques. Each week a different technique was facilitated, building on the previous week as the series progressed. The main objective was to demonstrate an aggregate increase in resilience as seen by pre- and post-survey scores based on an evidence-based resilience tool.

Some were skeptical when this program began. Many NHLs had reported using other types of wellness exercises in the past and were unsure how this would be different. During the series, some shared they were using HeartMath techniques for personal challenges in their lives: chronic pain, caregiver fatigue, or work-life balance.

The evaluation feedback was overwhelmingly positive:

- "I feel better prepared going through stressful events knowing I have tools to help."
- "HeartMath techniques helped me build resilience both professionally and personally."
- "I learned that I am not always as resilient as I think . . . implementing the tools will make a positive difference."

HeartMath demonstrated an aggregate increase in resilience from baseline. Two participants were so moved, they have taken steps to become HeartMath certified trainers themselves. Based on this program, techniques like HeartMath can be effective tools at increasing resilience in NHLs, further supporting the literature that utilizing programs like this have an overall positive effect on healthcare worker resilience. By prioritizing these tools, the overall workforce can be more resilient, and a strengthened organization can meet the needs of the community more effectively and compassionately.

Like most wellness exercises, these techniques, while simple, take practice. To be most effective, resilience techniques need to be incorporated into daily life so that when a challenge develops, you can easily pull one of these techniques from your resilience toolbox. You can't help anyone if you don't help yourself first, so remember to take a HeartMath moment.

References

Goldfisher, A. M., Hounslow, B., & Blank, J. (2014). Transforming and sustaining the care environment. *Global Advances in Health and Medicine*, *3*(Suppl. 1), BPA11. https://doi.org/10.7453/gahmj.2014.BPA11

HeartMath. (2021a). *Health professionals*. https://www.heartmath.com/health-professionals/heartmath-interventions-certification-program-001/

HeartMath. (2021b). *HeartMath*. https://www.heartmath.com/

HeartMath. (2021c). *Quick Coherence technique*. https://www.heartmath.com/quick-coherence-technique/

HeartMath. (2021d). *The science of HeartMath*. https://www.heartmath.com/science/

Makwana, N. (2019). Disaster and its impact on mental health: A narrative review. *Journal of Family Medicine and Primary Care*, *8*(10), 3090–3095. https://doi.org/10.4103/jfmpc.jfmpc_893_19

National Centers for Environmental Information. (2021). *Billion-dollar weather and climate disasters*. https://www.ncdc.noaa.gov/billions/

Rushton, C. H., Batcheller, J., Schroeder, K., & Donohue, P. (2015). Burnout and resilience among nurses practicing in high-intensity settings. *American Journal of Critical Care*, *24*(5), 412–420. https://doi.org/10.4037/ajcc2015291

Preparing for Disasters and Public Health Emergencies

Zenobia Harris, DNP, MPH, RNP
Past President and Diversity Representative, Association of Public Health Nurses

The overall ability of our national public health system that works daily to coordinate the protection and promotion of health for everyone in our local communities across this nation must become a priority for us all. Although the COVID-19 pandemic has exposed flaws in the systems of healthcare available in the US, it is not the only health crisis we have dealt with in America in our recent past. Each time we are confronted with and respond to a national health crisis—the 1918 influenza epidemic, the polio outbreak of the 1940s, the HIV/AIDS outbreak of the 1980s, the COVID-19 pandemic—tremendous differences in health outcomes related to race, income levels, housing, educational levels, employment status, and other demographics are revealed, often to our collective shame (Roberts, 2009).

During the influenza epidemic of 1918, African Americans experienced disproportionate case rates of disease and had to contend with legally sanctioned physical and psychological violence, segregation, and a system of Black labor abuse known as *peonage*. Racism played out in the relegation of African Americans to poorly trained providers and inferior hospitals, schools, and housing. It was reflected in the scientific racism of that time, which did not recognize the basic humanity of people of color when disease contact tracing and care was carried out (Gamble, 2010).

During the first days of the AIDS epidemic of the 1980s, an inadequate response occurred to address the torrent of death experienced by those affected by this disease (Brier, 2009). Although the AIDS epidemic was allowed to spread due to pathetic governmental response and discrimination against the populations most affected by the epidemic (Bennington-Castro, 2021), the activism of AIDS victims, health professionals, and other concerned citizens led to the development of promising treatment options.

The ongoing public health epidemic of violence in our society receives social attention but inadequate political action. An often-discussed side epidemic within the larger gun violence debate is the unacceptable rate of police-inflicted deaths experienced by people of color and the gun-related deaths experienced by young African American males in America (Frazer et al., 2018). Using data from the Centers for Disease Control and Prevention (CDC), the Johns Hopkins Center for Gun Violence Solutions reported that, in 2020, Black males between the ages of 15 and 34 constituted 38% of all people in the US who were victims of gun homicide—despite representing only 2% of the total population (2022).

From my experience, public health has ranked low on the nation's financial priorities list since our health focus shifted from an emphasis on containment of infectious disease in often-overwhelmed urban centers and under-resourced rural communities to a focus on financially lucrative chronic disease diagnosis and treatments. In recent decades, public health funding was awarded based on the extent of the public health crisis. What usually happens is when there is no health crisis, public health support and funding is reduced, which ensures that we are ill-prepared for the next crisis. The US public health system has been severely weakened by years of budget cuts and underfunding and lack of administrative development. This became clear during the onset of the COVID-19 pandemic.

State and local public health funding has been reduced by 16% or more over the past 10 years. Federal funding for emergency preparedness and response programs administered by the CDC has been cut by over 50% over the past decade, according to Trust for America's Health (2021).

To respond to current and future public health threats and emergencies more efficiently and effectively, the adequacy of funding for basic public health services—epidemiological surveillance, contact tracing, outreach, health education, immunization administration and tracking, HIV/AIDS and sexually transmitted infection treatment, reproductive health services, and food and water supply monitoring—has to be assured so that all communities have access to these vital services.

Unfortunately, the way we respond to these varying health outcomes in our communities has not significantly changed enough over the years to lead to the eradication of persistent health disparities in racial and ethnic minorities in the US (Mahajan et al., 2021). Communities of color and immigrant communities often receive more exposure to pollution in the air they breathe, the water they use, and the land they exist on because they live near sources of pollution such as interstate highways, factories, landfills, oil and gas industry work fields, airports, and military training facilities (Borunda, 2021).

In supplying care to individuals plagued by poor health outcomes, we must approach care looking at the population's access to care and targeted interventions such as testing. The societal and environmental exposure they must contend with as they live their lives—exposures that they often see as inescapable given the inadequate resources at their disposal regarding housing, job types, and educational opportunities—lead to the perpetuation of inequalities in health and personal safety (National Heart, Lung, and Blood Institute, 2022).

We must use the unique community outreach and engagement tools and relationships of the public health sector to develop epidemiological systems needed to define, address, and bring an end to the gun and interpersonal violence epidemic in our society (Belkin & McCray, 2019). Public health nurses can play a major role in providing support to communities as they work toward strategies that address local needs and prevention activities (Evans & Bufka, 2020).

The public health nursing leaders of today are being called upon to engage in advocacy for our profession at the national, state, and local institutional levels. We must develop and guard a strong public health nursing infrastructure to supply foundational public health services in all communities regardless of race, creed, or color.

As emergency funds from the Cares Act are being distributed across the US, nurses must engage in advocacy on behalf of the communities we serve to ensure that core public health services and supports are made available in all communities, especially those communities where our most marginalized citizens are forced to live and work due to historical discrimination.

References

Belkin, G., & McCray, C. (2019). Thrive NYC: Delivering on mental health. *American Journal of Public Health, 109*(S3), S156–163. https://doi.org/10.2105/AJPH.2019.305040

Bennington-Castro, J. (2021). *How AIDS remained an unspoken—but deadly—epidemic for years.* HISTORY. https://www.history.com/news/aids-epidemic-ronald-reagan

Borunda, A. (2021). *The origins of environmental justice—and why it's finally getting the attention it deserves.* National Geographic. https://www.nationalgeographic.com/environment/article/environmental-justice-origins-why-finally-getting-the-attention-it-deserves

Brier, J. (2009). *Infectious ideas: U.S. political responses to the AIDS crisis.* University of North Carolina Press. http://www.jstor.org/stable/10.5149/9780807895474_brier

Evans, A., & Bufka, L. F. (2020). The critical need for a population health approach: Addressing the nation's behavioral health during the COVID-19 pandemic and beyond. *Preventing Chronic Disease, 17,* 200261. http://dx.doi.org/10.5888/pcd17.200261

Frazer, E., Mitchell, R. A., Nesbitt, L. S., Williams, M., Mitchell, E. P., Williams, R. A., & Browne, D. (2018). The violence epidemic in the African American community: A call by the National Medical Association for comprehensive reform. *Journal of the National Medical Association, 110*(1), 4–15. https://doi.org/10.1016/j.jnma.2017.08.009

Gamble, V. N. (2010). "There wasn't a lot of comforts in those days": African Americans, public health, and the 1918 influenza epidemic. *Public Health Reports, 125*(3_suppl.), 113–122. https://doi.org/10.1177/00333549101250s314

Johns Hopkins Center for Gun Violence Solutions. (2022). *A year in review: 2020 gun deaths in the U.S.* https://publichealth.jhu.edu/gun-violence-solutions

Mahajan, S., Caraballo, C., Lu, Y., Valero-Elizondo, J., Massey, D., Annapureddy, A. R., Roy, B., Riley, C., Murugiah, K., Onuma, O., Nunez-Smith, M., Forman, H. P., Nasir, K., Herrin, J., & Krumholz, H. M. (2021). Trends in differences in health status and health care access and affordability by race and ethnicity in the United States, 1999–2018. *JAMA, 326*(7), 637. https://doi.org/10.1001/jama.2021.9907

National Heart, Lung, and Blood Institute. (2022). Health disparities and inequities. https://www.nhlbi.nih.gov/science/health-disparities-and-inequities

Roberts, S. K. (2009). *Infectious fear: Politics, disease, and the health effects of segregation.* The University of North Carolina Press.

Trust for America's Health. (2021). *The impact of chronic underfunding on America's public health system: Trends, risks, and recommendations, 2020.* https://www.tfah.org/report-details/publichealthfunding2020/

Learning Lessons From COVID-19: Upstream Fishing to Mend Downstream Implications

Hope Williamson-Younce, DNP, ACNP-BC, CCNS, CEN
Deputy Corps Chief, US Army Nurse Corps

Nurse leaders, you are the decisive element. The global nursing workforce was estimated as being 27.9 million nurses in 2019–2020 (World Health Organization, 2020). Arguably, the voices and actions of nurses play a crucial role in preparing communities for disasters and public health emergencies. The COVID-19 pandemic has exposed vulnerabilities in the nation's ability to handle a national-scale crisis (Healthcare Leadership Council, 2021). The unprecedented devastation from COVID-19 and evolving nationwide threats warrant our collective relook on how we operationalize future disasters and public health emergencies.

I will provide insight and practical application from lessons elucidated by the literature review and COVID-19 pandemic to address upstream turbulence while identifying opportunities for success in future disasters and public health emergencies. Thinking upstream was first introduced into nursing in 1990 to highlight the importance of advancing broad and context-rich perspectives of health for reducing health inequities by redirecting actions further up etiologic pathways and by putting emphasis on economic, political, and environmental health determinants (Butterfield, 2017). You, as the most trusted profession, have a moral obligation to get upstream and Plan-Do-Check-Act (PDCA) to mitigate the bodies being carried downstream in the social currents of health inequity (American Society for Quality, 2022):

- **Plan:** Through multisector, multidisciplinary stakeholder engagement across government agencies, state, tribal, and industry to identify the problem or opportunity and implement the best solution.

- **Do:** Identify potential solutions and test them on a small scale.

- **Check:** Study the results to ensure you are getting the desired outcomes.

- **Act:** Implement the solution and continue to look for ways to improve.

Similarly, prior to the COVID-19 pandemic, a PDCA-like framework and large-scale training exercise was implemented to achieve a high state of readiness among military health personnel from geographically dispersed installations around the world, which prepared the unit for an unprecedented, rapid response in support of COVID-19 relief efforts. As the Hospital Commander of one of the first Army Field Hospitals activated by the Department of Defense in March 2020, at the outset of the COVID-19 pandemic, transparent communication, cross-sector collaboration, maintaining a high state of readiness, and unity of effort proved vital to mission success. Nurse leaders can make a difference by engaging strategically upstream and leading from wherever they are. During the COVID-19 pandemic, diverse multidisciplinary US military teams were deployed to where they were needed most, to work side by side with their civilian partners (see Figure 6.2). They integrated into hospitals and communities and provided patient care, behavioral health, religious support, and medical supplies to diverse populations.

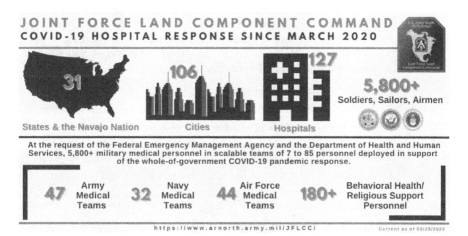

Figure 6.2 Joint Force Land Component Command.
US Army graphic by Lauren Padden, US Army North Public Affairs, 2022.

While the US military and nongovernmental agencies were able to provide much needed support, it is also important to honor the context of social determinants of health (SDOH), especially homes, workplaces, and local communities that received limited support. If one is to fully understand upstream as well as downstream, societal and structurally perpetuated norms that reinforced health disparities must be addressed (Butterfield, 2017). Let us consider the SDOH and upstream factors when striving for health equity across the local, state, and national levels, which are integral to improving disaster and public health emergency preparedness post-COVID-19. The conditions in which we are born, live, learn, work, and play—known as SDOH—have a profound impact on health, risk, opportunities available to practice healthy behaviors, and quality-of-life outcomes and expectancy. SDOH can be categorized into five domains (Healthy People 2030, n.d.):

- **Economic stability:** Safe housing, transportation, and neighborhoods
- **Healthcare access and quality:** Healthcare equity
- **Education access and quality:** Literacy skills, job opportunities, and income
- **Neighborhood and built environment:** Clean air and water; access to nutritious foods; physical activity opportunities; dismantling of racism, discrimination, and violence
- **Social and community context:** Family, friends, and support systems

Subsequently, the National Dialogue for Healthcare Innovation: Framework for Private-Public Collaboration on Disaster Preparedness and Response report comprises practical and actionable recommendations to strengthen our nation's response for future health crises to include strategies that nurses and federal, state, and private sector leaders can utilize to strengthen preparedness, resilience, response, and recovery (Healthcare Leadership Council, 2021):

- Equity and access issues must be proactively monitored and built into all phases of preparedness and response.
- Planning, coordinating, and collaborating must represent the perspectives of marginalized populations and diverse communities and be inclusive of racial and ethnic minorities, the uninsured, and people with disabilities.
- Stakeholders and health agencies should develop measures to track progress in improving equity and disparities during a public health emergency, building on the Centers for Disease Control and Prevention's COVID-19 Response Health Equity Strategy (Healthcare Leadership Council, 2021).
- Legislation and regulatory reform should enable rapid response capabilities in areas such as medical licensure portability, telehealth accessibility, and quick access to PPE stockpiles.

In closing, world events are sobering and, moreover, are a national call to action to enable nurses everywhere to band together and courageously forge the future. Often overlooked from a boots-on-the-ground experience, upstream policies should be codified to include embedded behavioral health and religious support services for frontline healthcare workers and first responders. Public health emergencies will become more frequent and severe; nevertheless, they can be handled more effectively with enhanced preparedness, beginning with the government at all levels and the private sector acting now, while lessons from COVID-19 are still being learned (Healthcare Leadership Council, 2021).

References

American Society for Quality. (2022). *What is the Plan-Do-Check-Act (PDCA) cycle?* https:// asq.org/quality-resources/pdca-cycle

Butterfield, P. G. (2017). Thinking upstream: A 25-year retrospective and conceptual model aimed at reducing health inequalities. *Advances in Nursing Science, 40*(1), 2–11. http://doi. org/10.1097/ANS.0000000000000161

Healthcare Leadership Council. (2021). *National dialogue for healthcare innovation: Framework for private-public collaboration on disaster preparedness and response.* https://www.hlc.org/wp-content/uploads/2021/01/disaster_preparedness_report-FINAL.pdf

Healthy People 2030. (n.d.). *Social determinants of health.* US Department of Health and Human Services, & Office of Disease Prevention and Health Promotion. https://health. gov/healthypeople/priority-areas/social-determinants-health

US Army North. (2022). *Joint forces land component command hospital support to COVID-19 response.* https://www.arnorth.army.mil/JFLCC/Covid-19-Response

World Health Organization. (2020). *State of the world's nursing 2020: Investing in education, jobs and leadership.* https://apps.who.int/iris/bitstream/hand le/10665/331673/9789240003293-eng.pdf

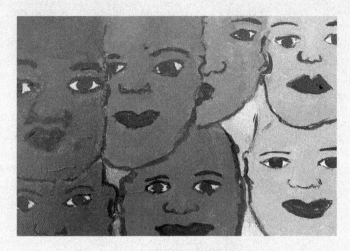

Face of Disparity

I am the face of disparity
I am right before you
You do not see me
Lost within statistics
Although, I am present
Fully aware of my situation
Alone, afraid, feelings of despair
Wondering what is happening to me
Will I be, OK?
I pretend not to care
I pretend to be strong
Illness shows my vulnerability
I wish I could keep my fear in the shadows
I have dreams, goals, potential
My culture gives me inner strength
I do not want illness to cause my failure
I need you to guide me
Fill me with knowledge
Help me live, laugh, love myself
Help me survive

Poetry and artwork by Lucinda Canty, PhD, CNM, FACNM
Associate Professor of Nursing, University of Massachusetts Amherst

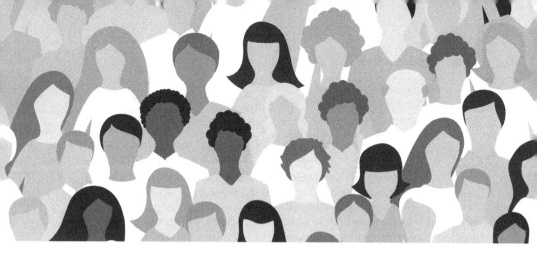

7 Innovation and Entrepreneur-ship

In This Chapter

- Technology as a Health Equity Lever

- Empowering Nurses to Own Our Pivotal Role in Advancing Technology, Innovation, and Entrepreneurship for Health Equity and Healthcare Transformation

- The Benefits of Nurse-Led Innovation and the Barriers to Overcome

- Technology Improvements to Promote Digital Health Equity

- Innovation Approaches to Increasing Equity and Decreasing Harm

Nurses possess the insight to improvise when resources are scarce, and that improvisation is appropriately viewed as innovation, especially since these nurse-initiated solutions improve health outcomes. Additionally, nurses lend their talents to the improvement of technology and move industries forward through entrepreneurship. As the world moves forward in the battle against disease, discrimination, and disparities, nurse ingenuity has the power and reputation to positively influence technology—from electronic health records to social media. We have a duty to disrupt the inequities perpetuated through, by, and because of technology (or lack thereof) that uphold and reinforce health inequities. And as nurses, we are perfectly poised to do so.

Consider the following questions as you read the essays about health equity and innovation and entrepreneurship:

- In what ways can technology perpetuate health inequities?
- How can nurses leverage their skills to become successful entrepreneurs?
- How can technology play a role in improving health outcomes?
- How do biases in technology affect health equity?
- Describe nursing innovations that promote health equity.

Technology as a Health Equity Lever

Shawna Butler, MBA, RN
Nurse Economist, Healthtech Specialist
Host, *SEE YOU NOW* podcast

Technology and digital connectivity have become a powerful, measurable determinant of health, education, opportunity, and prosperity—something of a public utility—almost like oxygen. They are so utterly essential to many parts of contemporary lifestyles, infrastructure, and economies. And by all accounts—surveys, reports, trends, and expert opinion—technology will become even more prevalent, running ambiently and continuously in every aspect of our waking and sleeping lives. According to the Pew Research Center, 42% of Americans say they have used technology in a way that has helped them personally be more independent or improve their quality of life (Strauss, 2020).

The year 2020 and the COVID-19 pandemic mark an important inflection point when healthcare learned with certainty that technology, tech-enabled people, and devices make it possible to accomplish big, complex, transformational projects—and accomplish them safely, swiftly, and effectively (Slotkin et al., 2021). COVID-19 also served as a forcing mechanism where we relied mightily, in some instances exclusively, on technology to respond to the health crisis and as well as enable a swift pivot to a remote, digital-first approach to our ongoing, non-crisis care, accomplishing in months what had previously taken years to achieve. It was during this sudden shift that healthcare also experienced, at scale and with unusual immediacy, the glaring realities, consequences, and inequities of the digital divide—the gap between those who have affordable access, skills, and support to effectively engage online and those who do not—and the critical importance of digital inclusion and equity (Close the Gap Foundation, 2022; National Digital Inclusion Alliance, 2022). Millions of Americans don't have access to broadband at home, and many more lack basic digital literacy skills.

Pointing its finger at the many inequities in our health, education, and social programs, the COVID-19 public health crises—like other pandemics before—provided a rare moment and opportunity to deeply reflect on our health equity performance, priorities, and definitions (Snowden, 2019). Health equity, as defined by physician, epidemiologist, and anti-racism activist Camara Jones, is "the assurance of the condition of optimal health for all people"—that health equity should be seen as a process rather than a final outcome (National Academies of Sciences, Engineering, and Medicine, 2019). COVID-19 health data and evidence across a wide range of metrics confirmed significant, distressing, and addressable disparities (Health Equity Tracker, 2022). The stories, lived experience, and activism ushered in the need for a health justice reckoning, mindset, and innovation agenda with a determination to fix that which has driven health disparities and steer directly to health equity (Network for Public Health Law, 2020). And nurses were—and are—uniquely positioned and prepared to be the engineers of technology-driven health equity. Prior to and throughout the pandemic, there are multiple instances where nurses used technology to design solutions addressing health needs while intentionally reducing disparities.

Nurses used the power of technology for building contact tracing teams, deploying chatbots as symptom checkers, and to provide education, medication reminders, schedule vaccinations, and health screenings, manage symptoms of depression and anxiety, and more (City of New York, 2022). Chatbots broaden access to people with disabilities, transportation challenges, language barriers, or work and living situations where in-person support is not an option. Nurses built virtual platforms and businesses on them to provide maternal and newborn care addressing the growing number of maternity care deserts and the extreme racial disparities in maternal and newborn mortality in the US (Baby Live Advice, 2022); telepsychiatry services as the need for mental health services skyrocketed (Lavender, 2022); and COVID-19 screening in homeless shelters, hard-to-reach places, and hardly-reached populations (Nurse Disrupted, 2022; Raths, 2021). Innovating at the intersection of diabetes, disparities, and digital health, nurses prescribe remote monitoring and wearable devices to track and share blood pressure, heart rate, glucose levels, weight, sleep patterns, physical activity, location, and movement to help patients manage chronic conditions (University of Utah Health, 2022). Nurses are using technology to reach and care for patients in an interesting and growing mix of conditions.

Prior to 2020, we were experiencing the beginnings of the consumerization of healthcare where technology, consumer preference, and business models were evolving and improving access and accessibility to quality, convenient, affordable healthcare (Deloitte, 2021; Sarasohn-Kahn, 2019). Sensors, data, AI algorithms, predictive analytics, virtual reality, and health apps were playing a major role in this directional shift and adoption. Using data and technology, people were able to make better health choices; nurses had far better real-time insights into populations' and individuals' health and could better manage conditions and panels of patients and provide highly targeted, personalized, timely health promotion and services. We saw billions of dollars invested in retail nurse-led primary care services, chronic condition management services, and healthcare startups focusing on digital health solutions and delivery models (Landi, 2022).

In hindsight, however, it appears healthcare was following and responding to the digital economy technology being built, and which tech-savvy consumers were rapidly adopting. Following, rather than leading, may have contributed to our disparities in connected healthcare access. Tech companies are known for their fast-paced innovation cycles. Healthcare, understandably conservative, is not. People on the margins may pay the price for this conservative stance. Using technologies to overcome or prevent barriers to healthcare is not a new concept, but COVID-19 accelerated their adoption and revealed just how easy it is to leave behind people without digital access, literacy, or devices in the rush toward connected, digital-centric healthcare. While there is boundless potential and a promise of technology being a democratizing force in healthcare—a lever for health equity—there is also a tremendous peril that our unevenly distributed technologies and infrastructure, and incomplete, biased data and algorithms, will accelerate and widen our existing health disparities and likely create new ones. When aligned with health equity, the promise of technology and the aim of digital inclusion can ensure that those with less purchasing power, autonomy, or some form of disability will not be left out of a world that offers infinite possibilities. If we are serious about eliminating the persistent racism and inequities in health, access, and care that contribute to poor outcomes and experiences for marginalized, vulnerable, and historically under-resourced communities, then nurses must, as they have throughout history, enthusiastically lead the way in cultivating technology and digital competencies for creating this preferred future of health equity.

References

Baby Live Advice. (2022). *Telehealth solutions for moms & babies*. https://babyliveadvice.com/

City of New York. (2022). *NYC test and trace*. https://www.nycservice.org/organizations/index.php?org_id=3772

Close the Gap Foundation. (2022). *Digital divide*. https://www.closethegapfoundation.org/glossary/digital-divide

Deloitte. (2021). *Road to next*. https://www2.deloitte.com/content/dam/Deloitte/us/Documents/audit/ASC/Roadmaps/us-auditq4-road-to-next-december-8th-edition.pdf

Health Equity Tracker. (2022). *Investigate rates of COVID-19*. https://healthequitytracker.org/exploredata

Landi, H. (2022). *Global digital health funding skyrockets to $57.2B with record cash for mental health, telehealth*. Fierce Healthcare. https://www.fiercehealthcare.com/digital-health/digital-health-startups-around-world-raked-57-2b-2021-up-79-from-2020#:%7E:text=In%20the%20U.S.%2C%20digital%20health,according%20to%20the%20report's%20findings

Lavender. (2022). *Your online psychiatry and therapy office*. https://www.joinlavender.com/

National Academies of Sciences, Engineering, and Medicine; Health and Medicine Division; Division of Behavioral and Social Sciences and Education; Board on Children, Youth, and Families; Roundtable on the Promotion of Health Equity; Forum for Children's Well-Being: Promoting Cognitive, Affective, and Behavioral Health for Children and Youth; Keenan, W., Sanchez, C. E., Kellogg, E., & Tracey, S. M. (2019). *Achieving behavioral health equity for children, families, and communities: Proceedings of a workshop*. National Academies Press.

National Digital Inclusion Alliance. (2022). *Definitions*. https://www.digitalinclusion.org/definitions/

Network for Public Health Law. (2020). *Health justice: Empowering public health and advancing health equity*. https://www.networkforphl.org/news-insights/health-justice-empowering-public-health-and-advancing-health-equity/

Nurse Disrupted. (2022). *Home*. https://www.nursedisrupted.com/

Raths, D. (2021). *Startup 'pair team' bolsters work of community health centers*. Healthcare Innovation. https://www.hcinnovationgroup.com/policy-value-based-care/medicare-medicaid/article/21250981/startup-pair-team-bolsters-work-of-community-health-centers

Sarasohn-Kahn, J. (2019). *HealthConsuming*. Think-Health LLC.

Slotkin, J. R., Murphy, K., & Ryu, J. (2021). How one health system is transforming in response to Covid-19. *Harvard Business Review*. https://hbr.org/2020/06/how-one-health-system-is-transforming-in-response-to-covid-19

Snowden, F. (2019). *Epidemics and society: From the Black Death to the present*. Yale University Department of History. https://history.yale.edu/publications/epidemics-and-society-black-death-present

Strauss, M. (2020). *Four-in-ten Americans credit technology with improving life most in the past 50 years*. Pew Research Center. https://www.pewresearch.org/fact-tank/2017/10/12/four-in-ten-americans-credit-technology-with-improving-life-most-in-the-past-50-years/

University of Utah Health. (2022). Can social and family networks improve our health? https://uofuhealth.utah.edu/newsroom/news/2022/02/social-networks.php

Empowering Nurses to Own Our Pivotal Role in Advancing Technology, Innovation, and Entrepreneurship for Health Equity and Healthcare Transformation

Elizabeth M. Perpetua, DNP, RN, ACNP-BC, ANP-BC, ARNP, FACC
Founder, Empath Health Services, LLC
Affiliate Instructor, Department of Biobehavioral Health and Informatics
University of Washington School of Nursing
Adjunct Professor, School of Health Sciences and School of Nursing
Seattle Pacific University

Consider your answer to this question: What important truth do few people agree with you on (Thiel & Masters, 2014)? For me, a first-generation Filipina-American and second-generation nurse, the best answer comes from a place of honesty, courage, and vulnerability.

There's no such thing as just a nurse. Nurses are leaders. Nurses are innovators. We are uniquely positioned for entrepreneurship.

"The best innovation is created by diversity of thought, opinion, insight, background, and culture. Nurses are natural innovators, creating solutions to alleviate human suffering based on their diverse experiences. The greatest healthcare technologies will be invented and informed by nurses; it is our time to lead. Carpe Diem!"

—Rebecca Love, BS, MSN, RN, FIEL
Chief Clinical Officer, IntelyCare

Empowerment begins with owning our story (Brown, 2010). Nursing is the largest and most trusted healthcare workforce in the US (Gallup, 2021; National Academies of Sciences, Engineering, and Medicine [NASEM], 2021). We have a pivotal role in the acceleration and implementation of every new health technology and therapy. We are on the front lines of healthcare, in each touchpoint of clinical operations, responsible for delivering and monitoring nearly every intervention that touches patients. Nurses are imperative to achieving the Quintuple Aim (Gallup, 2021): ensuring access to care, increasing cost effectiveness, and improving patient and team outcomes and experience. Transforming healthcare with innovation, technology, and entrepreneurship will not happen without the leadership and contributions of nurses.

No, these bold words did not feel like mine at the start. I felt safe and comfortable saying I am a short brown nurse just doing my job. I helped bring to patients many different medications, devices, and treatments, and patients lived longer and enjoyed a better quality of life. You have done this too. Because you are a nurse.

When products or processes did not work, my colleagues and I improved them. Early in my career in critical care, our solutions literally included tape and tongue depressors. In later leadership roles, we helped design new clinical pathways and standards of care. The prime example of this in my specialty is nursing's role in the rapid dispersion of transcatheter therapy for valvular heart disease, closing the typical 18-year gap from FDA approval to mainstream practice to mere months through dynamic coordination and systems of care (Balas & Boren, 2000; Nundy et al., 2022; Perpetua et al., 2019). In the COVID-19 pandemic, nurses are tasked to do more with fewer resources than ever before and as equitably as possible. I expect you have creatively solved the seemingly impossible many times. Because you are a nurse, you are an innovator.

Along the way I learn. I became an administrative leader, research investigator, professor of nursing leadership and role identity, and board member. I founded a technology-enabled consulting practice and built web-based applications to support this work. I was mentored and became a mentor. As scary and audacious as it felt, I brought to life ideas about products and services with the aim of helping many patients and teams. Why? Because I am a nurse. And why not? Nursing's professional role identity encompasses competencies inherent to accelerating innovation and promoting entrepreneurship (American Association of Colleges of Nursing, 2020).

To actualize the vision of health equity in the *Future of Nursing 2020-2030* report, nurses must be personally and professionally prepared and empowered to communicate about what we know, who we are, and what we do, which includes advancing technology, innovation, and entrepreneurship. Yes, we must address systemic factors contributing to health inequity and create the infrastructure to formally instruct nurses in innovation and entrepreneurship (NASEM, 2021). Yet our call to action begins within, to bring our own silence to voice, to know and own our unique story as individuals and as a profession. We are then better positioned to dismantle the power distance, hierarchy, and historical-cultural context that allows health inequity and disparity to persist. Here I offer for your consideration an image and a script to reflect upon your own stories.

Figure 7.1 provides an exercise in reflective practice which invites nurses to consider professional competencies and functions inherent to our role uniquely positioning us as innovators and entrepreneurs. Walking through the script may bring new, empowering language to the specific examples we already have or want to create in our lives. We build up these strengths as we progress in our journey and our role identity expands: Nurse Innovator (top left); Nurse Entrepreneur (bottom left). Sometimes fear can prevent us from embarking upon something new or unknown, even when we are the best suited to do so. Viewing this image as concentric rings (bottom right) may also serve as a reminder that as we grow and expand in our professional journey, our core role identity as providers to patients brings us strength and alignment.

Owning our story powerfully integrates the deeply personal with the universal. May we create the culture and conversation that unites us in our common humanity: courageous, vulnerable, and compassionate as we uplift one another, ensuring nurses are at every table where decisions are made about healthcare. Leadership, innovation, and entrepreneurship are not aspirational but integral to what we do, teachable and available to us. Because we are nurses.

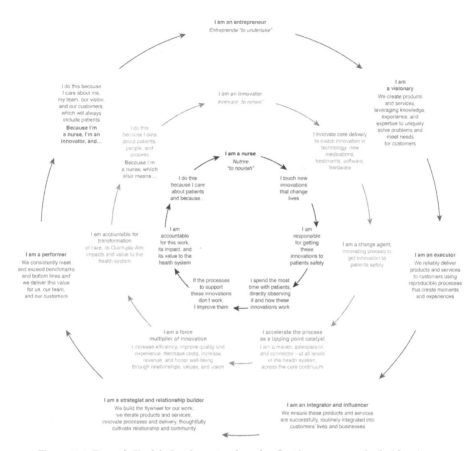

Figure 7.1 Empath Health Services storyboard reflection on nurses' role identity as innovators and entrepreneurs.

References

American Association of Colleges of Nursing. (2020). *Essentials of nursing practice*. https://www.aacnnursing.org/Portals/42/AcademicNursing/pdf/Essentials-2021.pdf

Balas, E. A., & Boren, S. A. (2000). Managing clinical knowledge for health care improvement. *Yearbook of Medical Informatics, 1*, 65–70. PMID: 27699347.

Brown, B. (2010). *Gifts of imperfection*. Hazelden Information & Educational Services.

Gallup. (2021). Annual honesty and ethics of professions poll 2021. https://news.gallup.com/file/poll/388700/220112HonestyEthics.pdf

National Academies of Sciences, Engineering, and Medicine. (2021). *The future of nursing 2020–2030: Charting a path to achieve health equity.* National Academies Press. https://nam.edu/publications/the-future-of-nursing-2020-2030/

Nundy, S., Cooper, L. A., & Mate, K. S. (2022, February 8). The quintuple aim for health care improvement: A new imperative to advance health equity. *JAMA, 327*(6), 521–522. https://doi.org/10.1001/jama.2021.25181

Perpetua, E. M., Clarke, S. E., Guibone, K. A., Keegan, P. A., & Speight, M. K. (2019). Surveying the landscape of structural heart disease coordination: An exploratory study of the coordinator role. *Structural Heart, 3*(3), 201–210. https://doi.org/10.1080/24748706.2019.1581962

Thiel, P., & Masters, B. (2014). *Zero to one: Notes on startups, or how to build the future.* Crown Business.

The Benefits of Nurse-Led Innovation and the Barriers to Overcome

Jennifferre Mancillas, BSN, RN, RNC-NIC
Co-Founder & Chief Operating Officer, Lumify

Nurses understand the disparities that patients and families face and often become the connective tissue between them and the healthcare system. With this understanding, nurses have the unique opportunity to create nurse-led innovations resulting in sustainable solutions that are both practical and personal and improve equity across the continuum of care. Importantly, unless nurse-led innovations are encouraged and fostered within the healthcare system, these opportunities to elevate the nursing profession and improve care will go unrealized. Common barriers for nurses in getting more involved with the work of innovating, and ideas to address the barriers include:

- Having a lack of direction:
  - Utilize a framework to solve the problem at hand, including the nursing process or design thinking. These processes will provide you with structure for next steps and help you to create and implement a more cohesive and well-rounded solution.
  - Access your organization's intellectual property and copyright policies. These policies provide guidance on expectations for you as the innovator, as well as provide you with potential resources.

> *"Our organizations must promote a culture of empathy, openness, and respect with diversity and inclusion. In the tech world, this means nurses are part of the design, development, and deployment of health technology solutions—as they bring a perspective that is essential to person-centered care."*
>
> Molly K. McCarthy, MBA, RN
> Managing Director, US Provider/Plans and Chief Nursing
> Officer, Microsoft

- Knowing who to talk to:

  - Build interdisciplinary relationships within your organization, such as those working in materials distribution, IT, and quality/safety. These relationships will assist you in navigating the resources available to you within your healthcare system. It is also a great way to catalyze innovation systemically.

  - Identify your organization's shared governance committees. These committees often work to create change through policy and procedure; finding a committee who can assist you in implementing your solution can be key in moving your innovation forward.

  - Find your champions. These people can be your fellow co-workers, supervisors, members of administration, or even community partners—anyone who will encourage your pursuit of innovation and help you to stay motivated.

There is a steady climb of nurses who are choosing to take their innovation further or utilize their skill sets outside of an organization and become entrepreneurs. Having nurses at the forefront of businesses focused on improving healthcare and supporting the healthcare workforce is a necessity. Nurses understand the needs of the communities they serve and the patients they care for intimately; as a result, they are capable of advocating for health equity and shaping the future of healthcare through the businesses they create. However, despite this vantage point, nurses who choose entrepreneurship will face unique challenges:

- Understanding how to start a business and utilizing your resources.

  - Online: YouTube, YC Startup School, Google, and more

  - Books: *The Lean Startup*, by Eric Ries (2014); *Zero to One*, by Peter Thiel and Blake Masters (2014); *7 Habits of Highly Effective People*, by Stephen Covey (2004)

- LinkedIn. People are often willing to help where they can and lend advice.

- Lean into the people within your network who are strong in the areas you are not and learn from them.

- Balancing working at the bedside and entrepreneurship.

  - Access and read through your organization's intellectual property and copyright policies. Having a clear understanding of who holds ownership of your business and/or product is important.

  - Allow for self-care. Working your scheduled shifts and using your days off to grow your business is not sustainable unless you find time to care for yourself.

- Challenging the perception for those outside of healthcare on the role of a nurse.

  - Remember that most startups fail because they struggle to reach product market-fit. As a nurse you understand the market you are building for better than most.

  - Show up in the spaces where non-nurse entrepreneurs are and own your knowledge.

  - Connect with other entrepreneurs and build up those relationships.

One of the fastest growing areas of technology is healthtech; subsequently we are beginning to see technology incorporated into nursing practice via enhancements to electronic health record systems, application-programming interfaces to support clinical care, and more sophisticated tech-enabled simulations for healthcare providers. In addition to tech being interwoven into nursing practice, nurses are proving themselves capable of creating tech solutions on their own in ways that resonate with users and meet the needs of patients; however, having a limited background in computer science does present challenges. Here are a few ways to work through the potential barriers:

- Use a "connect first, code next" approach. This means more time spent with users, resulting in a greater understanding of their needs and the build of a better product.

- Use contractors to fill the void of a technical lead while recruiting.

- Lean into your network and find a technical founder to advise on best practices to project manage technical contractors.

- Stay gritty and resourceful to gain traction and continue to build forward.

Nurses challenge the status quo within healthcare everyday by their innovation of practice and product. As versatile as the nursing profession is, a forward-thinking mindset can be incorporated into every pathway of nursing and be used to reform healthcare, improve patient care, and support the healthcare workforce. Encouraging and supporting nurse-led innovation is how we work towards improved health equity.

References

Covey, S. R. (2004). *The 7 habits of highly effective people: Restoring the character ethic*. Free Press.

Ries, E. (2011). *The lean startup: How today's entrepreneurs use continuous innovation to create radically successful businesses*. Crown Business.

Thiel, P., & Masters, B. (2014). *Zero to one: Notes on startups, or how to build the future*. Crown Business.

Technology Improvements to Promote Digital Health Equity

Mary Joy Garcia-Dia, DNP, RN, FAAN
Program Director, Nursing Informatics, Center for Professional Nursing Practice,
Corporate Nursing
New York-Presbyterian

As a nurse informaticist and a Filipino immigrant, I was acutely aware of the importance of data transparency during the recent COVID-19 pandemic. Our community was impacted disproportionately as the mortality rate for Filipino-American nurses was 30% higher than other nurses during the height of the pandemic (National Nurses United, 2020). Notably, the CDC did not separate Filipino data from that of Asians, non-Hispanic (Centers for Disease Control and Prevention, 2022). Dr. Norma Lang's quote, "If you can't name it, you can't practice it, you can't teach it, you can't pay for it, you can't research it, you can't put it into public policy" (Clark & Lang, 1992), resonated with me during these tumultuous events.

According to Kalyanaraman Marcello (2022), the deficient collection of standardized, disaggregated COVID-19 data at the state and county level has masked community-wide disparities that limited English-proficient, vulnerable communities of color have experienced. The invisibility of Asian Americans and other people of color in conversations about policy needs are traced to the lack of research specific to their experience. The cumulative underrepresentation in research studies leads to the vicious cycle of the lack of data that feeds the model minority myth, which suggests that Asians do not suffer economic or health disparities compared to whites.

Nurses have a critical role in capturing quality information and data as these drive the decision-making process for patient care, health systems' financial and clinical operations, and population health. Within the nursing informatics' domain, our clinical expertise and understanding of workflow processes drive the system design and build of clinical applications. From enterprise-wide electronic health records to stand-alone physiologic monitoring, surveillance systems, and point-of-care devices, nurses collect and contribute to the accumulation of big data. This increased access to data opens the opportunity to engage with underserved patients. Unfortunately, the lack of broadband access widens the digital divide for poor populations and those that reside in rural areas (Crawford & Serhal, 2020).

Nursing's influence in promoting health equity in the development of digital health solutions can minimize potential bias in machine learning algorithms using electronic health record (EHR) data. Gianfrancesco et al. (2018) identified sources of bias in EHR data and how this can affect marginalized populations. For example, missing data such as ethnicity, spoken language, primary written language, or patients not identified by algorithms can lead to misinterpretation resulting in inaccurate analyses and outputs. Smaller sample size can lead to underestimation. Miscalculation and measurement affect the quality of care due to implicit biases related to factors such as sex, age, and race. Gianfrancesco et al. (2018) looked at the process and provided approaches to minimize biases when implementing machine-learning algorithms:

- Overreliance on automation
    - Ensure interprofessional approach and engagement.
    - Conduct follow-up studies to ensure meaningful results.
- Algorithm based on biased data
    - Select training and testing sets and identify target population.
    - Build and test algorithms in a diverse healthcare system.
    - Include social determinants of health, race/ethnicity, and language in the variable.
    - Test algorithms for potential discriminatory behavior throughout data processing.
    - Develop feedback loops to monitor and verify output and validity.
- Nonclinical meaningful algorithms
    - Focus on clinically important improvements in outcomes rather than strict performance.
    - Impose human values in algorithms at the cost of efficiency.

The implementation of emerging technologies and innovation can potentially deepen existing inequities and create additional barriers. Rodriguez et al. (2020) noted that patient portal usage lags among underserved populations, including patients of racial/ethnic minoritized groups, limited English proficiency, low socioeconomic status, older age, and low literacy. Nurses can push for literacy metrics in designing mobile apps and patient portals to accommodate diverse patient populations and be cognizant of cultural, literacy, and linguistic needs. Using a sociotechnical approach, system designers can create conditions or tools to overcome health inequities by engaging with patients. The user-centered design approach understands and evaluates users, tasks, context, and environment. The inclusion of accessible design features and user-friendly navigational interfaces can minimize frustration and remove barriers. Nurse informaticist specialists can advocate in pushing for the revision of the Culturally and Linguistically Appropriate Services standards in incorporating equity in digital health tools.

Additionally, digital technology plays an increasingly important role in the healthcare industry with the recent growth of high-tech devices such as exercise trackers, heart monitors, and other mobile devices and smartphones. Brewer et al. (2020) noted existing bias with wearable technology such as the smartwatch with an acceptable error range in capturing vital signs. Manufacturers rely on green light sensors through a process called photoplethysmography to detect heart rate, respiration temperature, and calculate the body mass index. The report demonstrates less reliability in accurately monitoring heart rates in people of color, especially those with darker skin tones. The failure to engage with diverse populations during the development phase could lead to downstream health disparities and mistrust in technology. There is a need to systematically consider digital health equity framework and integrate digital health policies, strategies, and programs to ensure that potential health inequities are identified when collecting data, creating cultural/linguistic contents, and/or monitoring health equity outcomes for potential system bias.

Being that the goal is to expand information sharing and increase data portability as the patient moves from different phases of care, opportunities exist in using predictive modeling to increase a patient's self-efficacy in taking control and managing health concerns or illness. For example, based on family history, behavioral patterns, disease process, compliance with medications, risk factors, and physical activity, data analytics can project what the overall health status would look like for a newly diagnosed 35-year-old diabetic patient in three to five years. Thus, an early intervention plan of care and targeted outcomes can be designed to engage the patient proactively. Nursing informatics services [NIS] and APNs can create partnerships through a health coach model that supports the patient's clinical and information management needs. This can be facilitated through a hybrid interaction that is flexible enough to accommodate face-to-face visits or virtual visits. As communities continue to deal with COVID-19 spread, the use of other telecommunication tools (Zoom, Snapchat, WeChat, Google, basic landline telephone) will need to be considered, depending on the patients' familiarity with the tools, geographic location, time zones, and broadband connections.

Regardless of technology use and adoption, the human element of caring is an integral part of nursing practice and patient engagement. The value and contribution of nursing informatics professionals will continue to spread beyond geographic lines, expanding globally and virtually.

References

Brewer, L. C., Fortuna, K. L., Jones, C., Walker, R., Hayes, S. N., Patten, C. A., & Cooper. L. A. (2020). Back to the future: Achieving health equity through health informatics and digital health. *JMIR Mhealth Uhealth, 8*(1), e14512. https://doi.org/10.2196/14512

Centers for Disease Control and Prevention. (2022, April 12). *COVID data tracker.* https://covid.cdc.gov/covid-data-tracker

Clark, J., & Lang, N. (1992). Nursing's next advance: An internal classification for nursing practice. *International Nursing Review, 39*(4), 109–111, 128.

Crawford, A., & Serhal, E. (2020). Digital health equity and COVID-19: The innovation curve cannot reinforce the social gradient of health. *Journal of Medical Internet Research, 22*(6), e1936. https://doi.org/10.2196/19361

Gianfrancesco, M. A., Tamang, S., Yazdany, J., & Schmajuk, G. (2018). Potential bias in machine learning algorithms using electronic health record data. *JAMA Internal Medicine, 178*(11), 1544–1547. https://doi.org/10.1001/jamainternmed.2018.3763

Kalyanaraman Marcello, R., Dolle, J., Tariq, A., Kaur, S., Wong, L., Curcio, J., Thachil, R., Yi, S. S., & Islam, N. (2022). Disaggregating Asian race reveals COVID-19 disparities among Asian American patients at New York City's public hospital system. *Public Health Reports, 137*(2), 317–325. https://doi.org/10.1177/00333549211061313

National Nurses United. (2020). *Deadly shame: Redressing the devaluation of registered nurse labor through pandemic equity.* https://www.nationalnursesunited.org/sites/default/files/nnu/graphics/documents/1220_Covid19_DeadlyShame_PandemicEquity_WhitePaper_FINAL.pdf

Rodriguez, J. A., Clark, C. R., & Bates, D. W. (2020). Digital health equity as a necessity in the 21st century Cures Act era. *Journal of American Medical Association, 323*(23), 2381–2382. https://doi.org/10.1001/jama.2020.7858

Innovation Approaches to Increasing Equity and Decreasing Harm

Marion Leary, MSN, MPH, RN
Director of Innovation, University of Pennsylvania School of Nursing

Jonathan Zhu, BSN student, University of Pennsylvania School of Nursing

In the era of pandemics, burnout, and staffing shortages, innovation can sometimes be overlooked by healthcare systems that may not understand how it can be used to empower nurses, improve health equity, and decrease harm.

When defined, *innovation* is the "solving of pressing problems using rigorous methodological approaches infused with creativity and risk-taking. [Innovation] embraces clinical, social, technological, educational, policy, and process change" (Leary et al., 2022, p. 86). True innovation, though, requires that solutions be co-created with and are accessible by the community for whom the problem affects, with the goal of improving health outcomes.

Multiple innovative approaches can be used in health and healthcare to collaboratively create solutions and center the needs of end-users. Human-centered design is one such approach to problem-solving in which end-users are continuously involved and consulted for their input and experience (IDEO Design Thinking, n.d.). Nurses are ideal candidates for engaging in this form of innovation because they focus on patient-centered care. Many innovation approaches have been developed based on the human-centered design framework, including design thinking, equity-centered design, and liberatory design.

Design thinking is a methodological approach used in human-centered design that centers on the needs of those for whom the application is designed (Design Thinking for Health, 2022; IDEO Design Thinking, n.d.). Design thinking is an iterative process generally consisting of five stages: empathize, define, ideate, prototype, and test. The empathy stage is foundational throughout the entire process and allows the designers to understand the users' needs intrinsically and extrinsically. Empathy uses in-situ interviews and observations to understand the problem from the stakeholder's perspective, in the environment where the problem is occurring (Design Thinking for Health, 2022; Dining et al., 2018).

Equity-centered design is an innovation practice that incorporates elements of design thinking but asks the design team to reflect on the "actions, emotions, insights and impact" the design process has on the end-users (d.School, 2022a). The basis of equity-centered design is the involvement of under-resourced communities throughout the design process to remove power differences that lead to oppression, exclusion, and health inequity (Equity Design Thinking, 2022).

Cultivating a culture of equity requires a robust framework, and this approach emphasizes the importance of nurturing humility, integrating historical perspectives, and addressing power dynamics (Srivastava, 2021).

Finally, *liberatory design* is an approach that aims to help designers develop self-awareness throughout the design process in order to break away from traditions that preserve inequity. In the process, power is shifted from the designers to those affected by the problem (d.School, 2022b; Liberatory Design, 2021). Liberatory design is built on the beliefs that systemic racism and inequity can be redesigned, equitable design requires participation from those affected by inequity, and the complex nature of challenges should inform the design approach (Liberatory Design, 2021).

Underlying these approaches are the principles of *design justice*, where design is used to deconstruct structural inequality and liberate communities from oppressive and exploitive systems to heal, empower, and support communities (Costanza-Chock, 2020). With a design justice lens, designers and innovators examine how pre-existing systems and design impact the distribution of risk among groups (Costanza-Chock, 2018). This perspective encourages decentering the designers and centering the voices of the communities directly affected to address their most significant challenges and needs more accurately (Costanza-Chock, 2020).

At the University of Pennsylvania's School of Nursing (Penn Nursing), we provide this innovation education using a two-pronged approach of traditional classroom learning and active, hands-on learning to infuse these innovation approaches throughout the curriculum.

For traditional learning, we teach a variety of classes focused on innovation and health design including our introductory class, Innovation in Health: Foundations of Design Thinking. This is an interdisciplinary course that is open to students across the university (Karwat et al., 2021). In this course, students learn about the design thinking process by focusing on health and healthcare problems by collaborating in teams with key stakeholders to create solutions. Students are exposed to design justice principles throughout the course and reminded to engage with their stakeholders during the entire design process, capturing their lived experiences and centering their wants and needs. Recently, a summer institute for Africana Studies at Penn included a course called Innovation in Health Equity. This course examined the structural causes of health inequity and looked at how innovation and activism converged to advance health outcomes in historically marginalized communities of color (Brooks Carton, 2021).

For active-learning opportunities, a new initiative at Penn centered around social justice principles is the Community Collaboratory for Co-Creation (Penn4C). Penn4C is a collaboration between Penn Nursing and the Penn School of Engineering and Applied Sciences and seeks to facilitate and co-create projects with marginalized communities based on their needs. Students, along with faculty, put design principles learned in the classroom into practice by co-creating with community members to create solutions to improve health, well-being, and safety (Community Collaboratory for Co-Creation, n.d.). Additionally, students and faculty are encouraged to participate in nurse-led hackathons, accelerators, and other active-learning innovation challenges that focus on decreasing health inequity and increasing co-collaboration and human-centered solutions (Kagan et al., 2021).

Nurse-led innovation is an exciting and rapidly expanding area of interest which can help bring about tremendous improvements in health outcomes. Ultimately though, as designers, researchers, and clinicians, we must always consider who is involved in the design process, who is harmed, and who benefits (Equity Design Thinking, 2022). When nurses are educated on the innovation approaches of human-centered design, equity-centered design, liberatory design, and the principles of design justice, it will lead to more nurses using these approaches in practice and creating more equitable innovations that reduce health disparities, promote equity, decrease harm, and improve health outcomes.

References

Brooks Carton, J. M. (2021). *Innovation for health equity*. University of Pennsylvania.

Community Collaboratory for Co-Creation. (n.d.). *Designing technology for social justice & health*. https://www.penn4c.org/

Costanza-Chock, S. (2018). *Design justice: Towards an intersectional feminist framework for design theory and practice*. Proceedings of the Design Research Society.

Costanza-Chock, S. (2020). *Design justice: Community-led practices to build the worlds we need*. The MIT Press.

Design Thinking for Health. (2022). *Design thinking: Introduction*. https://designthinkingforhealth.org/the-course/introduction/

Dining Zuber, C., & Moody, L. (2018). Creativity and innovation in health care: Tapping into organizational enablers through human-centered design. *Nursing Administration Quarterly, 42*(1), 62–75. https://doi.org/10.1097/NAQ.0000000000000267

d.School. (2022a). *Equity-centered design framework*. https://dschool.stanford.edu/resources/equity-centered-design-framework

d.School. (2022b). *Liberatory design*. https://dschool.stanford.edu/resources-collections/liberatory-design

Equity Design Thinking. (2022). *The equity design educational series*. University of Pittsburgh. https://pittequitydesignthinking.org/

IDEO Design Thinking. (n.d.). *What's the difference between human-centered design and design thinking?* https://designthinking.ideo.com/faq/whats-the-difference-between-human-centered-design-and-design-thinking

Kagan, O., Littlejohn, J., Nadel, H., & Leary, M. (2021). Evolution of nurse-led hackathons, incubators, and accelerators from an innovation ecosystem perspective. *OJIN: The Online Journal of Issues in Nursing, 26*(3), 3. https://doi.org/10.3912/OJIN.Vol26No03Man03

Karwat, A., Richmond, T. S., & Leary, M. (2021). Transition of a collaborative in-person health care innovation course to online learning. *Journal of Nursing Education, 60*(5), 298–300. https://doi.org/10.3928/01484834-20210420-12

Leary, M., Villarruel, A. M., & Richmond, T. S. (2022). Creating an innovation infrastructure in academic nursing. *Journal of Professional Nursing, 38*, 83–88. https://doi.org/10.1016/j.profnurs.2021.12.005

Liberatory Design. (2021). *Liberatory design: mindsets and modes to design for equity.* https://liberatorydesign.com

Srivastava, A. (2021, August 10). *What is equity-centered community design?* Bootcamp UX Design. https://bootcamp.uxdesign.cc/what-is-equity-centered-community-design-4a49cb55003f

Love Remains

Music & Lyrics Written by Tad Worku

Tad Worku is a songwriter, singer, speaker, and nurse practitioner. His music is available via most music streaming services. You can find out more at tadworku.com.

Back Story: I wrote this song after experiencing the death of my first patient. The patient had come into the ED alert and oriented but quickly declined through my shift. When I got home, I needed to process through the idea of hope, faith, and love in that moment. I wrote this song as a response to that experience

V1
I've seen life, slowly fading away
I've seen death, try and take it away
I've seen pain, drop a tear on a face
But in all, I've seen
Love Remains, Love Remains

I've seen hope, from the depth of despair
I've seen peace, coming out from nowhere
I've seen grace, wash the deepest of stains,
In all, I've seen, Love remains

CHORUS
You see people always told me just wait and see
When you get a little older the world will be
Darker like the stain on a window pane
But I can see, through the stain
Love Remains, Love Remains

CHORUS REPEAT
You see people always told me just wait and see
When you get a little older the world will be
Darker like the stain on a window pane
But I can see, through the stain
Love Remains, through the stain
I can see through the stain
Love Remains, Love Remains

OUTRO
Love Remains, Love Remains, ooh ooh
Love Remains, Love Remains
Love Remains, Love Remains, ooh ooh ooh
Love Remains, Love Remains

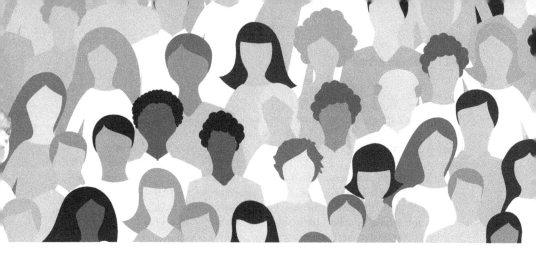

8 Nurse Well-Being: Compassion for Self and Others

In This Chapter

- Restoring Respect, Compassion, and Equity by Fostering Nurse Well-Being

- Resiliency, a Double-Edged Sword: Improving the Culture and Climate of Nursing

- Crossing the Cultural Chasm Between Mental Health Stigma and Care-Seeking Behaviors in Nursing

- Self-Care Is Not Selfish

Nurses have experienced burnout, posttraumatic stress disorder, and even death in the battle against COVID-19. While none of this is new to those who are experienced in the field, the pandemic brought these issues, along with many important others, to the forefront. It is imperative for us to care for nurses and to teach nurses to care for themselves so that they can continue their honorable work. In this chapter, the focus is on the importance of nurse well-being and its potential to promote positive health outcomes and equity. So often nurses are held in high esteem for their tremendous sacrifices, which is greatly appreciated; however, this positive view of sacrificial actions may encourage nurses to overlook or push through any physical and/or mental challenges they may be experiencing as a result. We encourage you to be cognizant of your own state of well-being and that of others and to get assistance for yourself and others. After all, how can we facilitate wellness when we are not well?

Consider the following questions as you read the essays about health equity and nurse well-being:

- What wellness and mental health resources are available where you learn and work?

- How can nurses contribute to the well-being of one another?

- What are concerns of nurses who may want to seek mental health services?

- What steps can be taken to reduce the negative impacts of mental health–related stigmas?

- How is the well-being, both mental and physical, of nurses directly related to patient/client care?

Restoring Respect, Compassion, and Equity by Fostering Nurse Well-Being

Cynda Hylton Rushton, PhD, RN, FAAN
Anne and George L. Bunting Professor of Clinical Ethics
The Johns Hopkins Berman Institute of Bioethics and the School of Nursing

The pandemic has brought into sharp focus the limits and profound consequences of the patterns of self-sacrifice within the profession and the structures that have created and reinforced oppressive and disproportionate burdens on nurses (Stokes-Parish et al., 2020). These realities parallel systemic societal patterns of gender inequality, broken trust, commodification, and disregard for the humanity of all persons. Intertwined with these realities in healthcare are the societal expectations of nurses to uphold their social contract without a corresponding responsibility of Americans to contribute to their own health and to extend the respect they expect for themselves to the nurses who are delivering care (Fry-Bowers & Rushton, 2021). Aggression and violent incidents against nurses are alarmingly high (El Ghaziri et al., 2021).

> *"As nurses, we cannot take great care of others unless we take good self-care; if not, we will need to take the time for illness later. For us to enhance health equity and promote the highest level of well-being in all populations, we must stop pouring from an empty cup. If you do not do it for yourself, do it for the people who love you and want you to be around for a long time to come."*
>
> –Bernadette M. Melnyk, PhD, RN, APRN-CNP, FAANP, FNAP, FAAN
> Vice President for Health Promotion, University Chief
> Wellness Officer, Dean and Helene Fuld Health Trust Professor of
> Evidence-Based Practice, College of Nursing,
> The Ohio State University

Creating and sustaining equity in healthcare delivery must include equitable investment in the humanity of nurses delivering it. Whether we are addressing questions of respect and equality at the bedside, in the community, or beyond, we cannot give what we do not have ourselves. When we are exhausted and depleted, it is difficult to access empathy or compassion or to muster the energy to invest in systemic change. We can lose sight of our purpose and meaning and become angry, sad, and disengaged. When we work in environments that do not foster our basic health, well-being, and integrity though priorities, processes, and structures, the detrimental consequences intensify and accumulate. Seeing our workforce through the lens of equity opens new avenues for addressing the symptoms and root causes of degraded well-being and links our efforts to the fundamental values of our profession. Just as the first provision of our Code of Ethics calls us to care for every person with respect and dignity for their personhood, so too is the same respect owed to nurses (American Nurses Association, 2015).

It is tempting to say that the system is the whole problem, but fixing the system is a partial solution—just as focusing only on individuals is a partial solution. It's not either/or—it must be both/and. Systems are comprised of people—we are the system (however we define it). When the people in the system are depleted and disengaged, meaningful and sustainable progress is unattainable. Likewise, when the system is not designed to support our fundamental well-being, resilience, integrity, and individual capacities to meet adversity, it becomes a continuous cycle of despair, disengagement, and dissonance. The solution is to synergize individual and systemic strategies to create the ecosystem that supports nurses in fulfilling their calling and purpose with compassion, rather than an environment of judgment and blame. When individuals and systems align their efforts, sustainable progress is possible.

Where Do We Begin?

Throughout my career I have listened to and borne witness to the challenges and the triumphs of nurses in different roles and specialties. Again and again, I have been inspired by their courage, compassion, commitment, and competence. How do we cultivate compassion and restore humanity in our profession and healthcare? How do we heal the wounds of the pandemic?

Why Compassion?

Compassion is a word often used to signal a feeling state associated with perceiving the suffering of others and being motivated to take action to relieve their suffering (Halifax, 2011). But compassion is more than a feeling state. It is a complex, emergent process, involving non-compassion elements, that produces principled, wise action (Halifax, 2012). This notion of compassion, described by Roshi Joan Halifax, goes beyond the typical characterization of compassion that is reduced to being "kind" or in limited supply, resulting in "compassion fatigue." Terms such as *compassion fatigue* are likely misapplied; studies suggest it is *empathy* rather than compassion that has become overwhelmed and fatigued (Klimecki & Singer, 2011). Terms like *compassion fatigue* inadvertently suggest that compassion is something to be avoided rather than cultivated. Such characterizations of compassion have the potential to undermine the power of compassion to transform ourselves and others and the central role of compassion in healing ourselves, our relationships, systems, and society.

Cultivating the Condition for Compassion to Arise

Halifax has developed a mnemonic, G.R.A.C.E., to reflect the elements necessary for compassion to emerge (Halifax, 2012, 2013). The elements of G.R.A.C.E. are:

1. Gather attention

2. Recall intention

3. Attune to self and others

4. Consider what will serve

5. Enact ethically

These simple, nonlinear, and emergent elements provide a scaffolding for application in different contexts but require ongoing practice to develop the architecture to support compassion in action.

Application of G.R.A.C.E. to Explore Self-Stewardship

The elements of G.R.A.C.E. can be applied to your well-being and self-stewardship. "Self-stewardship embodies a commitment to know oneself, to responsibly and mindfully manage one's personal resources, to recognize and compassionately respect one's limitations, and to choose actions that are wholesome and life affirming" (Rushton, 2018, p. 137). How can we be good stewards of our own resources and well-being? G.R.A.C.E. illuminates a path of self-stewardship grounded in compassion. The process creates the conditions for compassion to arise toward our own limitations and unmet expectations rather than animating old self-destructive patterns that undermine our well-being and integrity. When we resource ourselves with compassion, we are more likely to be able to extend compassion to others. This grounding supports us in showing up for our patients, families, and communities in a more balanced way and can create the foundation for compassion to arise in our relationships with others. It offers the foundation for acting from a place of restored agency, to choose rather than react, and the fuel to address the issues of health equity that arise in our daily practice. The G.R.A.C. E. process is a valuable resource to restore our integrity and foster our moral resilience when moral adversity arises (Rushton, 2018). The elements of G.R.A.C.E. can be applied in myriad situations, especially those where conflict, uncertainty, or tension are present, as a means for discovering a path of compassionate action.

Investing in your well-being and wholeness creates the foundation for constructively engaging in system re-design and cultural change. When you have invested in self-stewardship, you can choose where you invest your energy, time, and talents. This doesn't suggest that fixing the system is your responsibility alone. Rather, investing in self-stewardship is an act of integrity that acknowledges to yourself that you are worthy and deserving of your investment regardless of what the system does or does not do. But without such investment and clarity, it is easy to lapse into feeling victimized and powerless to choose or act.

The elements of G.R.A.C.E. can also be used as a resource in addressing systemic contributions to degraded well-being. Using compassion as a lens for system change opens avenues for exploring solutions to old problems with new eyes. Consider what might arise if all the members of leadership applied the process of G.R.A.C.E. when making budget allocations, setting staffing standards, or investing in new programs. It's possible that with a stable attention and nervous system, connecting to values and purpose and attunement to self and others would reveal new possibilities to consider and enact (Hougaard et al., 2021).

References

American Nurses Association. (2015). *Code of ethics for nurses with interpretive statements.* Author. https://www.nursingworld.org/coe-view-only

El Ghaziri, M., Johnson, S., Purpora, C., Simons, S., & Taylor, R. (2021). Registered nurses' experiences with incivility during the early phase of COVID-19 pandemic: Results of a multi-state survey. *Workplace Health & Safety.* Advance online publication. https://doi.org/10.1177/21650799211024867

Fry-Bowers, E. K., & Rushton, C. H. (2021, September 23). *Who will be there to care if there are no more nurses?* The Hastings Center. https://www.thehastingscenter.org/who-will-be-there-to-care-if-there-are-no-more-nurses/

Halifax, J. (2011). The precious necessity of compassion. *Journal of Pain and Symptom Management, 41*(1), 146–153. https://doi.org/10.1016/j.jpainsymman.2010.08.010

Halifax, J. (2012). A heuristic model of enactive compassion. *Current Opinion in Supportive and Palliative Care, 6*(2), 228–235. https://doi.org/10.1097/SPC.0b013e3283530fbe

Halifax, J. S. (2013). G.R.A.C.E. for nurses: Cultivating compassion in nurse/patient interactions. *Journal of Nursing Education and Practice, 4*(1), 121–128. https://doi.org/10.5430/jnep.v4n1p121

Hougaard, R., Carter, J., & Afton, M. (2021, December 23). Connect with empathy, but lead with compassion. *Harvard Business Review.* https://hbr.org/2021/12/connect-with-empathy-but-lead-with-compassion

Klimecki, O., & Singer, T. (2011). Empathic distress fatigue rather than compassion fatigue? Integrating findings from empathy research in psychology and social neuroscience. In B. Oakley, A. Knafo, G. Madhavan, & D. S. Wilson (Eds.), *Pathological altruism* (pp. 368–383). Oxford University Press.

Rushton, C. (2018). Conceptualizing moral resilience. In C. Rushton (Ed.), *Moral resilience: Transforming moral suffering in health care* (pp. 125–149). Oxford University Press.

Stokes-Parish, J., Elliot, R., Rolls, K., & Massey, D. (2020). Angels and heroes: The unintended consequence of the hero narrative. *Journal of Nursing Scholarship, 52*(5), 462–466. https://doi.org/doi:10.1111/jnu.12591

Resiliency, a Double-Edged Sword: Improving the Culture and Climate of Nursing

Martha A. Dawson, DNP, RN, FACHE, FAAN
13th President, National Black Nurses Association
Associate Professor, University of Alabama at Birmingham School of Nursing

For decades, nursing has supported a healthy work environment promoting an anti-bullying climate and non-violent patient-to-nurse interaction. More recently, *The Future of Nursing 2020–2030: Charting a Path to Achieve Health Equity* took a bold step to "call out" our profession to address racism in nursing (National Academies of Sciences, Engineering, and Medicine, 2021). This report mentioned the word *racism* over 90 times, indicating that as a profession, we must be willing to lead in this space as we address health inequities and improvement in population health.

I want to call my profession to action to have brave and curious conversations that are action-oriented to address racism through lived experiences of nurses of color without creating similar harm for our white colleagues. However, I ask my white colleagues to become active allies that are open to listening and learning.

The National Commission to Address Racism in Nursing (2021, p. 1) defines racism as "assaults on the human spirit in the form of actions, biases, prejudices, and an ideology of superiority based on race that persistently causes moral suffering and physical harm of individuals and perpetuates systemic injustices and inequities." Examination and reflection on Dr. King's quote and the commission's definition inform us of two concepts that are receiving a lot of discussions in the nursing space today: public health and resiliency.

Black supremacy is as dangerous as white supremacy, and God is not interested merely in the freedom of black men and brown men and yellow men. God is interested in the freedom of the whole human race and the creation of a society where all men will live together as brothers, and all men will respect the dignity and the worth of all human personality.

–Rev. Martin Luther King Jr., September 1960, DePauw University

First, some smart social scientist or academician decided that racism is a public health crisis. This statement can be dispelled with the definition of public health by the Centers for Disease Control and Prevention (2014). This leading body defines public health as the science of promoting and protecting the health of people by tracking, reporting, preventing, and responding to disease outbreak. Simply stated, nurses are people, not a disease, and when we experience racism, it does not impact the public health of the general population, but it causes moral suffering and physical harm to those who have to live this experience every day. This is why so many historically excluded nurses have to practice hyper-resiliency.

Resiliency as a concept has been used to describe nurses' response to stressful work environments, colleague relationships, the prolonged COVID-19 pandemic, and, more recently, addressing racism in the profession. There is a vast amount of literature and evidence addressing resiliency as a tool defining how people react to stressful situations or life adversities. Nursing is a rewarding career, but the very nature of the work has inherent stress, amplifies interpersonal interaction, and requires mental acuity. There is no debate that nursing as a profession requires resiliency. However, the million-dollar question is what percentage of stress and adverse events occurs externally or internally to the profession. For nurses of color, experiencing racism, professional isolation, inequity, and inequalities could cause them to have a heightened need to remain in a constant state of practicing resiliency, adding to their daily stress and affecting their mental health.

Great nurse leaders and scientists should explore the concepts of racism, resiliency, inequity, and inequality relative to nurse burnout, medication errors, turnover rate, and absenteeism. Nursing is a science-based and theory-enriched practice. Therefore, I invite nurse leaders to study theories of humanity, expectancy, equity, and organizational justice. These theories can and will help us address issues that are creating mental blocks and holding us back from acknowledging our past and forging a future as healthcare leaders. No, hiring a diversity, equity, and inclusivity dean will not address or solve our problems. Most of these roles do not have the power and influence to address leaders and the leadership teams' practices, organizational policies, and the distribution of resources and support. Stop trying to make me feel as if I "belong" and create a culture and climate where I know I belong. It is not just about awards, recognition, social events, and belonging; it is about me being my authentic, best self. Nursing needs an awakening, and change starts with leaders.

References

Centers for Disease Control and Prevention. (2014). *Introduction to public health in: Public Health 101 series*. https://www.cdc.gov/training/publichealth101/public-health.html.

Civil Rights Leader Rev. Martin Luther King Jr. Speaks on the DePauw Campus. (1960, September 5). DePauw University. https://www.depauw.edu/news-media/latest-news/details/33427/

National Academies of Sciences, Engineering, and Medicine. (2021). *The future of nursing 2020-2030: Charting a path to achieve health equity*. National Academies Press. https://nam.edu/publications/the-future-of-nursing-2020-2030

National Commission to Address Racism in Nursing. (2021). *Defining racism*. https://www.nursingworld.org/~4a0e54/globalassets/practiceandpolicy/workforce/commission-to-address-racism/final-defining-racism.pdf

Crossing the Cultural Chasm Between Mental Health Stigma and Care-Seeking Behaviors in Nursing

Charlene Grace Platon, MS, RN, FNP-BC
Director of Ambulatory Nursing, Stanford Health Care
Chief Executive Officer and Co-Founder, Fifth Window

The repeated surges of the COVID-19 pandemic have shown that the prioritization of nurses' mental health needs is more important now than ever before. However, stigmas toward individuals with mental illnesses are pervasive across the healthcare industry and serve as a major barrier to care-seeking behaviors (Knaak et al., 2017). Unfortunately, nurses and healthcare professionals are not exempt from the impacts of mental illness–related stigma. In a recent study, nurses and healthcare workers who reported suicidal ideations were more reluctant to seek help than healthcare workers without reported suicidal ideations (Kelsey et al., 2021).

> "Nurse leaders must fully own who they are, what they understand about themselves, and what they know, as this is foundational to grounded confidence and leadership. One can't pour from an empty cup—strong leadership demands a strong bedrock of self-care."
>
> –Eileen T. O'Grady, PhD, RN, NP-BC
> Author, *Choosing Wellness: Unconventional Wisdom for the Overwhelmed, the Discouraged, the Addicted, the Fearful, or the Stuck*

Stigma is a complex construct and represents one fragment of a nurse's or health-care professional's decision to pursue mental health services. However, stigmati-zation in healthcare occurs simultaneously on intrapersonal, interpersonal, and structural levels (Knaak et al., 2017). On a structural level, barriers preventing nurses from seeking care may include concerns regarding their career, confidenti-ality, and time-off approval to attend appointments. In addition, nursing licensure applications may include questions about mental health and can serve as a barrier for nurses seeking mental health treatment (Kelsey et al., 2021). There are addi-tional nuances of this stigma when looking through the contexts of our diverse multicultural communities.

To more fully grasp the nuances of healthcare stigma, it is important to discuss the definitions of both mental illness and mental health, two terms that are often used interchangeably. *Mental illness* refers to current or past psychiatric disorders that result in functional impairment (Alegria et al., 2010), whereas *mental health* is inclusive of an individual's emotional, psychological, and social well-being (Cen-ters for Disease Control and Prevention, 2021). When considering the diverse cultures within our organizations or communities, some families may exhibit sig-nificant reluctance in seeking mental health services, even with concerning signs of mental illness present.

As a Filipino American female who was born and raised in the United States by two immigrant parents and who has pursued my entire career in the healthcare industry, my own reluctance to seek mental healthcare services and disclose men-tal health challenges was two-fold. The dichotomies of my personal and profes-sional lives shared the common theme of mental illness–related stigma, and this manifested as an overwhelming sense of shame and avoidance of mental health treatments. In various Asian communities, mental illnesses may be perceived as a reflection of flaws within the family. This shame can be amplified by the desire to conform to social norms, resulting in less likelihood to seek mental health services (Corrigan et al., 2014). In fact, various cultures view mental illness as "incurable" or "unresponsive to modern medical treatments" (Alegria et al., 2010, p. 49). As a result of this amplified shame that I personally experienced, I suffered in silence. During nursing school, I chose not to inform my professors or preceptors of my mental health struggles, even during the most challenging of times. Admittedly, I carried this behavior with me as I transitioned through various stages of my healthcare career, demonstrating the significant impact that stigma has played in my life.

Despite the complexities surrounding mental illness–related stigma, there are steps that can be taken to reduce the negative impacts of stigma for the diverse communities within the healthcare industry. Nevertheless, it is important to acknowledge that one solution does not fit all experiences. Sustainably reducing stigma will require addressing the perception of mental healthcare on multiple levels. At the individual level, providing stigma reduction training for all health-care employees can promote awareness of stigmas and their effects on one's own attitudes. Another best practice is the establishment of safe spaces or platforms placing individuals with the stigmatized conditions or behaviors at the core. On a structural level, anti-discrimination policies must be developed and enforced, as well as implementing reporting mechanisms within healthcare facilities (Nyblade et al., 2019).

Committing to the reduction of mental illness–related stigmas will benefit more than only the nurses and healthcare professionals who receive these mental health services. By reducing stigmas, there are potentials to improve workplace environments, quality of patient care delivery, and clinical outcomes of individuals living with stigmatized health conditions (Nyblade et al., 2019).

Today, there are still times in which I am reluctant to share my experiences and challenges with mental health. In fact, I have reflected on how different my life and career-related experiences may have been if stigma reduction strategies were embedded in my nursing journey at the very start. While I will never be able to comprehend what could have been, I am optimistic about the promotion of mental well-being among nurses and healthcare professionals, and what is yet to come.

References

Alegria, M., Atkins, M., Farmer, E., Slaton, E., & Stelk, W. (2010). One size does not fit all: Taking diversity, culture and context seriously. *Administration and Policy in Mental Health and Mental Health Services Research*, *37*(1–2), 48–60. https://doi.org/10.1007/s10488-010-0283-2

Centers for Disease Control and Prevention. (2021). *About mental health*. https://www.cdc.gov/mentalhealth/learn/index.htm

Corrigan, P. W., Druss, B. G., & Perlick, D. A. (2014). The impact of mental illness stigma on seeking and participating in mental health care. *Psychological Science in the Public Interest*, *15*(2), 37–70. https://doi.org/10.1177/1529100614531398

Kelsey, E. A., West, C. P., Cipriano, P. F., Peterson, C., Satele, D., Shanafelt, T., & Dyrbye, L. N. (2021). Original research: Suicidal ideation and attitudes toward help-seeking in U.S. nurses relative to the general working population. *American Journal of Nursing*, *121*(11), 24–36. https://doi.org/10.1097/01.naj.0000798056.73563.fa

Knaak, S., Mantler, E., & Szeto, A. (2017). Mental illness-related stigma in healthcare: Barriers to access and care and evidence-based solutions. *Healthcare Management Forum*, *30*(2), 111–116. https://doi.org/10.1177/0840470416679413

Nyblade, L., Stockton, M. A., Giger, K., Bond, V., Ekstrand, M. L., Lean, R. M., Mitchell, E. M. H., Nelson, L. R. E., Sapag, J. C., Siraprapasiri, T., Turan, J., & Wouters, E. (2019). Stigma in health facilities: Why it matters and how we can change it. *BMC Medicine*, *17*(25). https://doi.org/10.1186/s12916-019-1256-2

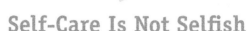

Self-Care Is Not Selfish

Maureen T. White, MBA, RN, NEA-BC, FNAP, FAAN
Executive Vice President & Chief Nurse Executive, Northwell Health

Launette Woolforde, EdD, DNP, RN, NEA-BC, NPD-BC, FAAN
Chief Nursing Officer, Lenox Hill Hospital, Northwell Health

While nurses have a long-standing history of serving the community, they are not immune to the same social determinants of health and factors that affect the well-being of the communities they serve. As nurses treat others in need of care, they often do so while dealing with their own struggles and challenges. Many health conditions that people experience are connected, either directly or indirectly, to their background, their historical experiences, and their physical and social environment. The COVID-19 pandemic exacerbated the long-standing disparities in care that exist and highlighted social and mental health issues that our populations, including nurses, endure. Day after day, nurses give so much of themselves as they care for others. In doing so, nurses and other healthcare providers often overlook their own physical and mental health needs. To provide sound care to others, it is critical that nurses pay particular attention to caring for themselves.

"Joy in Practice is a collaborative effort across UnitedHealth Group to bring together internal and external partners who are committed to reducing burnout and increasing professional joy. For example, we host 'Bonfires' to help clinicians refocus away from the negative stressors and *instead celebrate the good we have achieved. Connecting with others to exhale our stress and collectively inhale the renewed sense of purpose and meaning has been tremendous."*

–Mary Jo Jerde, MBA, BSN, FAAN
Senior Vice President, Center for Clinician Advancement,
UnitedHealth Group

Nurse Well-Being Increases Patient Well-Being

Nurse self-care is an essential ingredient in providing quality care to the communities we serve. Burnout and fatigue can contribute to feeling overwhelmed when providing care, making nurses more prone to committing medication and other errors, bypassing essential steps, or missing signs of changes in a patient's condition.

Highlighting the importance of self-care and offering programs to embed self-care into nurses' lifestyles and professional practice demonstrates an investment in the health of not only the individual nurse but also in the health of the patients they care for. By focusing on their own well-being, nurses can gain a deeper understanding of holistic care and are likely to carry this into their practice. Nurses who maintain their well-being may be able to cope with stressors more effectively and in turn demonstrate greater patience and empathy when supporting patients through their own struggles. Nurses may be more attuned to the importance of providing resources, support, and guidance which helps their patients balance their own well-being, thus contributing to broad improvements in health.

Nurse well-being can also translate into practice in ways that foster health equity. Self-care and well-being support mental clarity, centeredness, and mindfulness. This can help nurses better recognize health equity shortcomings in care planning and care delivery. Ideally, nurse well-being can contribute to nurses making recommendations that result in a more comprehensive treatment plan for their patients. This may include advocating for greater mental health support, social services, community programs, and more for their patients.

What Can Employers Do?

As healthcare organizations start to focus on their role and responsibility in health equity, population health, and wellness, they too should become a beacon for nurses in supporting them in caring for themselves. Healthcare organizations depend on nurses, and nurses should be able to depend on their healthcare organizations as well—not just as a place that they or other patients can turn to for treatment when they are sick, but also as a place that they as employees can turn to in order to prevent illness and maintain wellness.

Employers should create platforms that encourage and allow nurses to express what their well-being needs are. Business Employee Resource Groups (BERGs) are one way that organizations can achieve this. BERGs bring employees together based on commonalities or common interests, and BERG members identify ways in which they desire to be supported and support others. Knowing that the cumulative effect of unaddressed stressors can result in emotional and mental breakdown as well as physical deterioration and loss of quality of life, organizations can demonstrate support for nurses by creating entities dedicated to traumatic stress, recovery, and resiliency building. Stress First Aid is one such offering that can be provided to assist nurses as they navigate the realities and pressures of life

(US Department of Veterans Affairs, 2022). These programs strengthen coping mechanisms, teach stress reduction techniques, and provide much needed support. Employee health and wellness programs focused on exercise, nutrition, financial security, and family support services, for example, can also contribute to nurse well-being. Employee virtual walks such as a Walk to Paris, where teams come together to walk the number of steps it would take to travel from one location to Paris, are another option employers can offer. Chef challenges to develop easy to prepare and nutritionally healthy meals for the busy team member with competing priorities can also engage the workforce in self-care and well-being. Programs that provide financial education and advisement for short-term and future planning may also offer much needed resources for nurses' well-being balance. Similarly, family support programs that consider both child and elder care can prove invaluable in alleviating stressors.

However, one size does not fit all. Organizations need to take a multifaceted approach that centers on hearing the voices of and understanding the needs of their nurses.

Promoting Positive Health Outcomes and Health Equity

Nurses enter the profession to care for others; however, this very premise may contribute to nurses overlooking the need to care for themselves. As nurses become more in touch with their individualized self-care needs, this will translate into becoming more engaged and empathic in addressing the self-care needs of diverse populations. The first step in population health begins with the health of our caregivers, especially our nurses.

As the health needs of our nurses and caregivers evolve, so too must the health and wellness offerings to address their needs. Healthcare organizations need to be in tune with evolving their health and wellness offerings as new modalities arise and new programs develop. This is a dynamic process that has no finish line. The health of our society is inextricably linked to the health of our nurses and workforce.

Reference

US Department of Veterans Affairs. (2022). *Stress first aid: Manuals and resources for health care workers*. https://www.ptsd.va.gov/professional/treat/type/stress_first_aid.asp

Peace of Mind

Music & Lyrics Written by Tad Worku

Tad Worku is a songwriter, singer, speaker, and nurse practitioner. His music is available via most music streaming services. You can find out more at tadworku.com.

Back Story: In 2019, I went Per Diem in the ER after 5 years as a nurse. I had the opportunity to tour internationally and speak for hospital system executive summits, mission/vision conferences, and GALAs. I was booked for most of 2020 with my Grammy Award-winning team. On March 16th, 2020, everything got canceled. I wrote this song as I processed through all the changes and the fact that I would be dealing with COVID on the front lines.

V1

Time pass, fade away
Life changes in so many ways
You build your puzzle and you file away
Plans change but it will be okay
Plans change but it will be okay

Sometimes dreams fade
Left broken in so many ways
With all the pieces you finally see
All along you had a plan for me
All along you had a plan for me

CHORUS

So open my eyes help me to see the truth
That all my goodbyes
Brought me closer to you
All the fear inside
Circling my mind, help me to find
Give me peace of mind

V2

Tears fall fade away
Like shadows on a rainy day
I know the sun will always light 'em away
Rain comes but it will be okay
Rain comes but it will be okay

Some days, I'll need memories
Of laughter looking after me
I know the morning's coming after the night
Hold on cause it will be alright
Hold on cause it will be alright
Hold on cause it will be alright now yeah
Hold on cause it will be alright

CHORUS

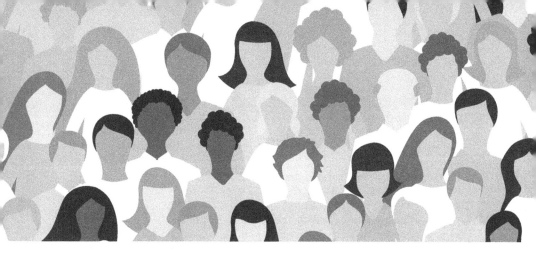

9 Global Stewardship

In This Chapter

- Nurses as Champions for Global Health Equity

- Nurses Caring for Their Communities Around the World

- Region of the Americas: Health Systems and Nursing

- Addressing the Worldwide Nursing Workforce Shortage: "There's no justice . . . just us"

- Global Stewardship: Reimagining the Adage "Think Global, Act Local" in the Post-Pandemic World—Every Nurse's Business

Even though we may live, work, and play thousands of miles from each other geographically, global travel and technology have essentially made us all neighbors. Culture and the ways in which we live our lives vary greatly around the world, but we all experience illnesses that are rarely unique to one individual. As such, this chapter considers the global perspective as it relates to health equity. This includes sharing and adapting best practices in health equity around the globe and understanding our global fit and responsibility to promote health equity. We recognize that health management and interventions should be tailored to and culturally appropriate for a specific community or population. However, because we are genetically more alike than different, we encourage nurses to become global citizens by sharing successful, evidence-based practices that advance health equity.

Consider the following questions as you read the essays about health equity global stewardship:

- How can nurses working where you live champion health equity globally?

- What are potential negative effects of ignoring the health outcomes of your global neighbors?

- How can nurses help mitigate health inequities perpetuated by racism and discrimination?

- What are examples of nursing-related solutions in foreign countries that may be applicable in your own country?

- What social structures or determinants facilitate health inequities around the world?

Nurses as Champions for Global Health Equity

Yvonne Commodore-Mensah, PhD, MHS, RN, FAAN, FPCNA
Associate Professor, Johns Hopkins University School of Nursing

As the largest healthcare workforce, nurses are well-poised to champion efforts to advance global health equity. Health equity, as a principle, is not limited by geographic boundaries, population, or condition. As such, regardless of where you find yourself in the world, you can advocate for equity in health access, services, and outcomes for all populations, especially those who are marginalized.

"The pandemic has starkly highlighted the world's lack of preparedness and ruthlessly exacerbated existing inequalities in our societies, yet alarmingly, we have seen nations retreat from multilateralism. There is no one-nation solution to any of the global health challenges that we face; we must work together and include health in all policies. In the next decade, it is the strength of our health systems that will determine both the health of people as well as the health of our economies and the safety and security of societies. Our global health workforce is both health and peace makers; their work is an expression of our humanity in practice, and their leadership is essential to a fairer, safer, and healthier world."

–Howard Cotton
Chief Executive Officer, International Council of Nurses

We need a health equity lens because there are pervasive and unjust health inequities worldwide. For instance, although life expectancy increased globally from 66.8 years in 2000 to 73.4 years in 2019, this improvement has not been experienced by most low- and middle-income countries (LMICs; World Health Organization [WHO], 2022b). While a person born in the United Kingdom or United States can be expected to live to be 81 years or 79 years respectively, their counterparts who are born in Lesotho, South Africa, or Mozambique will live to be 51 years and 58 years, respectively (WHO, 2022a). The factors that drive these stark differences in life expectancy include disparities in the burden of communicable and non-communicable diseases, healthcare resources, healthcare workers, and economic development, to name a few.

One of the most marginalized populations globally is migrants and refugees. Although migration is a global phenomenon, ongoing crises—including conflicts in Africa, the Middle East, Europe, and Latin America—climate change, and violence have contributed to the surge in migration. In 2020, over 281 million people were considered migrants, representing 3.6% of the global population (International Organization for Migration, 2019). Migrants and refugees often have limited access to education, healthcare resources, and employment opportunities, limiting their opportunity to attain optimal health. The WHO Global Action Plan on Promoting the Health of Refugees and Migrants 2019–2023 has established a comprehensive framework of priorities and guiding principles to promote the health of migrants and refugees (WHO, 2019), which includes policies and short- and long-term public health interventions to advance the health of migrants and refugees. Nurses should support this action plan and lend their voices to global policies that promote migrant and refugee health and address the unique lived experiences of these marginalized populations.

As the largest healthcare workforce globally, nurses are well-positioned to advance health equity and improve health locally and globally. The International Council of Nurses [ICN] has stressed that nurses play a pivotal role in serving as advocates for social justice and equity, resource allocation, access, and social and economic services (ICN, 2021). To contribute to global efforts to advance health equity, we must first address critical challenges in the nursing workforce in LMICs. While high-income countries have lower patient-to-nurse ratios, in LMICs, there is a dire shortage of nurses to manage the double burden of communicable and non-communicable diseases. The ICN has chronicled the global nursing shortage and challenges of filling the gap of 13 million nurses that are needed globally (ICN, 2022). Moreover, the burnout and heavy workloads that nurses experienced before the COVID-19 pandemic have been exacerbated by the ongoing global health emergency. Undoubtedly, the impact of the COVID-19 pandemic has been disproportionately experienced by nurses residing in LMICs. Although nurses around the globe have grappled with obtaining access to personal protective equipment to prevent the transmission of COVID-19, nurses in LMICs continue to work in unsafe conditions and without sufficient mitigation measures to avoid exposure to health hazards. To that end, nurses should advocate that governments protect the safety and wellness of all nurses in all settings. Investments in training, recruiting, and retaining nurses will strengthen health systems and fill critical gaps in care during the pandemic and beyond.

There is a unique opportunity for local to global collaborations among nurses in high-income countries with their counterparts in LMICs to advance their scope of practice, training opportunities, research and clinical practice, and educational partnerships. Although global partnerships between nurses in high-income countries and LMICs have increased recently, there are opportunities to evaluate the impact of these partnerships in improving health outcomes and narrowing health disparities (Nishimi & Street, 2020). Examples of successful global partnerships include the Botswana–American International Health Alliance, Toronto Addis Ababa Academic Collaboration, Nursing Faculty Development Programme, and the Maternal and Child Health Initiative (Nishimi & Street, 2020). These global partnerships, which include distance learning among nurses in LMICs, non-degree workshops, nurse faculty development programs, and collaborative curriculum development, are aligned with WHO's call for enhancing nursing education (WHO, 2011) and the *Future of Nursing 2020–2030: Charting a Path to Achieve Health Equity* report (National Academies of Sciences, Engineering, and Medicine, 2021). Recent experiences with the COVID-19 pandemic, the Ebola outbreak, Zika, and H1N1 underscore the importance of well-connected and well-resourced healthcare systems in addition to a robust supply of well-trained nursing workforce.

As we educate nurses for the future, we must emphasize that a nurse trained in Atlanta, Georgia; Bangkok, Thailand; or Brasília, Brazil is a global nurse steward. One who espouses the values of social justice, equity, courage, and resilience to tackle global health challenges in every corner of the world. One who upholds the intrinsic value of every person across the life span and promotes dignity in sickness and in health.

References

International Council of Nurses. (2021). *The ICN code of ethics for nurses*. https://www.icn.ch/sites/default/files/inline-files/ICN_Code-of-Ethics_EN_Web.pdf

International Council of Nurses. (2022). *The global nursing shortage and nurse retention*. https://www.icn.ch/news/greatest-threat-global-health-workforce-shortage-international-council-nurses-international

International Organization for Migration. (2019). *World migration report 2020*. https://worldmigrationreport.iom.int/wmr-2020-interactive/

National Academies of Sciences, Engineering, and Medicine. (2021). *The future of nursing 2020–2030: Charting a path to achieve health equity*. National Academies Press. https://nam.edu/publications/the-future-of-nursing-2020-2030

Nishimi, K., & Street, N. W. (2020). Nursing education partnerships between western high-income universities and non-governmental agencies and low-income local agencies: A scoping review of the literature. *Journal of Professional Nursing, 36*(3), 147–157. https://doi.org/10.1016/j.profnurs.2019.08.010

World Health Organization. (2011). *Transformative scale up of health professional education: An effort to increase the numbers of health professionals and to strengthen their impact on population health*. https://www.who.int/publications/i/item/transforming-and-scaling-up-health-professionals%E2%80%99-education-and-training

World Health Organization. (2019). *Promoting the health of refugees and migrants. Draft global action plan 2019–2023*. 72nd World Health Assembly.

World Health Organization. (2022a). *Global health expectancy: Life expectancy and healthy life expectancy*. The Global Health Observatory. https://www.who.int/data/gho/data/themes/mortality-and-global-health-estimates/ghe-life-expectancy-and-healthy-life-expectancy

World Health Organization. (2022b). *Life expectancy at birth (years)*. The Global Health Observatory. https://www.who.int/data/gho/data/indicators/indicator-details/GHO/life-expectancy-at-birth-(years)

Nurses Caring for Their Communities Around the World

Pamela F. Cipriano, PhD, RN, FAAN
President, International Council of Nurses
Professor of Nursing
University of Virginia School of Nursing

Nurses have always been at the forefront of helping marginalized populations thrive and have long believed that everyone should have access to quality, affordable healthcare known as "universal health coverage," or UHC, which has become a worldwide imperative. Ten years after the United Nations General Assembly endorsed UHC in 2012 and urged countries to work to achieve health for all, we're falling short of building the healthier world envisioned by 2030. Millions are forced into poverty from their personal spending on healthcare, and many more suffer without access to essential healthcare services. The 2021 campaign for UHC Day declared the theme, "Leave no one's health behind: invest in health systems for all." In tandem, the Human Rights Day's theme was, "Equality—Reducing inequalities, advancing human rights." While these are global goals, you play an important role helping achieve them.

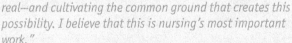

"How strange we humans are in our need to create the borders and walls that ultimately keep us captive in our own predispositions and prejudices. How sad this is when hope for humankind and the future for this planet lies with each of us reaching beyond those barriers, both imagined and real—and cultivating the common ground that creates this possibility. I believe that this is nursing's most important work."

–Marla E. Salmon, ScD, RN, FAAN
Professor of Nursing and Global Health,
University of Washington

The International Council of Nurses (ICN) has posted case studies about nurses caring for their communities to make the acts of nurses providing access to care more visible to the world. Over the past several years, numerous examples have illuminated how nurses are making a difference. Table 9.1 highlights ways that

nurses on every continent are bringing care to underserved populations and leveraging their work and research findings to change health policy and impact even
greater numbers of people. Many activities align with international campaigns to
address priorities of the United Nations and World Health Organization (WHO)
as well as country-level measures that support the same.

Table 9.1   Nurses Caring for Their Communities and Addressing Health Disparities

Country	Alignment With International Campaign-Specific Focus	Nursing Actions and Impact	Source for More Information
Canada	International Human Solidarity Day Palliative care for homeless living in poverty	PhD-prepared clinical nurse specialist introduced palliative care to people who otherwise would not have had access to this essential care.	https://www.icn.ch/news/international-nurses-day-2020-case-study-week-48
Uruguay	International Migrant's Day Culturally appropriate healthcare for migrants	Provide migrants access to culturally appropriate and acceptable healthcare as well as assistance with many social issues.	https://www.icn.ch/news/international-nurses-day-2020-case-study-week-47
Kenya	World AIDS Day Getting care to more people living with HIV, including access to retroviral therapy	Nurse-midwives provide care to marginalized populations, which is helping to decrease mortality (currently accounts for 29% adult deaths and 20% maternal mortality) and morbidity, including reduced hospital admissions for infections.	https://www.icn.ch/news/international-nurses-day-2020-case-study-week-45

continues

Table 9.1   Nurses Caring for Their Communities and Addressing Health Disparities   (cont.)

Country	Alignment With International Campaign-Specific Focus	Nursing Actions and Impact	Source for More Information
Spain	Raise public understanding and utilization of nurses	Family and community nurses educated public to boost health promotion and prevention uptake with earlier detection of health problems and control of noncommunicable diseases; helping increase UHC.	https://www.icn.ch/news/get-most-your-nurse-campaign-spain

We have learned that unless everyone is safe, no one is safe from direct and existential threats to health, whether they occur naturally or are man-made. In April each year, World Health Day focuses attention on creating healthy societies. The 2022 poignant theme "Our planet, our health" aligns with a dominant conversation about the urgency of addressing the effects of climate change, one of the greatest threats to health and prosperity. Nurses are working in coalitions to insist on climate justice that will help protect people from the many effects of disrupted ecosystems (see Figure 9.1). They are helping to mitigate the local effects while relying on national and global efforts to do more to change the conditions that threaten the planet.

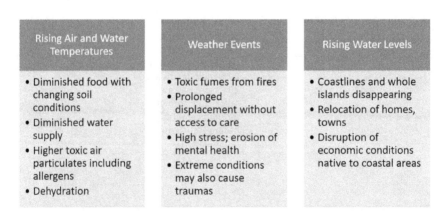

Rising Air and Water Temperatures	Weather Events	Rising Water Levels
• Diminished food with changing soil conditions • Diminished water supply • Higher toxic air particulates including allergens • Dehydration	• Toxic fumes from fires • Prolonged displacement without access to care • High stress; erosion of mental health • Extreme conditions may also cause traumas	• Coastlines and whole islands disappearing • Relocation of homes, towns • Disruption of economic conditions native to coastal areas

Figure 9.1 Ecosystems disrupted by climate change.

Addressing vaccine equity throughout the pandemic is an example of injustice borne out in many lower-income countries. Not only have health workers not been prioritized in some countries, but distribution of vaccine supplies occurred at highly variable rates, allowing many to be unprotected and potentially die at greater rates. ICN consistently and repeatedly advocated for vaccine prioritization of at-risk groups, including nurses and healthcare workers, as well as calling on governments to take immediate and sustained action to ensure equitable and unbiased access for all people through whatever means were needed in all countries.

Those least likely to be able to seek education and lucrative employment remain at a disadvantage and are more adversely affected by threats to physical and mental health. Gender inequity and racism plague almost every society, as women and minorities are held back by cultural practices and historic laws that prohibit them from realizing their potential. Additionally, individuals who identify as lesbian, gay, bisexual, transgender, and queer (LGBTQ) have experienced difficulty accessing the health system as well as cumulative stress from discrimination, stigma, and fear of violence, leading to higher rates of physical and mental health problems and poorer health outcomes (Medina-Martinez et al., 2021). Given the high burden of disease for those holding a gender identity and sexual orientation other than male/female binary gender and heterosexual, the National Institute on Minority Health and Health Disparities Health in 2016 designated sexual and gender minorities as a health disparity population for NIH research (Perez-Stable, 2016). Drivers of this inequality are described in Figure 9.2.

Two other areas of great concern that are threats to health equity are gender inequity and systemic racism. Both of these unfortunate realities are likely responsible for perpetuating many health disparities in countries where women and minorities are undervalued and more likely to endure lower socioeconomic status.

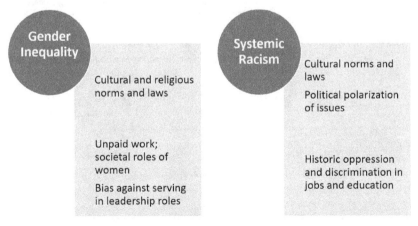

Figure 9.2 Restraints on gender and race.

In more subtle ways, women consistently are disadvantaged as they voluntarily or out of necessity take on unpaid domestic work that competes for their time every day. This is true in nursing and was supported as a key finding in the report *Delivered by Women, Led by Men: A Gender and Equity Analysis of the Global Health and Social Workforce* (WHO, 2019). Men enjoy more rapid ascent to leadership roles, described as a glass escalator, whereas women are disadvantaged by taking time out for childbirth and other household roles. In climate change as well, women are adversely affected as the ones who take primary responsibility for their families and must adapt to find food, water, care, and protective living conditions.

Health as a human right is an ambitious global goal that demands UHC, gender equity, and racial justice. Removal of legal, financial, social, and institutional barriers that restrict access to health services is an essential ingredient to achieving health equity. So, too, removal of racism as an obstacle to health equity brings us closer to health for all. You can help eliminate the public health crisis caused by racism by pursuing honest conversations and raising your voice when you see an injustice or discriminatory act that threatens someone's physical or mental health or access to care. We can't change the color of our skin, but we can choose to intervene to eliminate differences in care so that we can improve the health of our nation and the world.

References

Medina-Martínez, J., Saus-Ortega, C., Sánchez-Lorente, M. M., Sosa-Palanca, E. M., García- Martínez, P., & Mármol-López, M. I. (2021). Health inequities in LGBT people and nursing interventions to reduce them: A systematic review. *International Journal of Environmental Research and Public Health*, *18*(22), 11801. https://doi.org/10.3390/ijerph182211801

Pérez-Stable, E. J. (2016). *Director's message: Sexual and gender minorities formally designated as a health disparity population for research purposes.* Retrieved from https://www.nimhd.nih.gov/about/directors-corner/messages/message_10-06-16.html

World Health Organization. (2019). *Delivered by women, led by men: A gender and equity analysis of the global health and social workforce.* https://apps.who.int/iris/handle/10665/311322

Region of the Americas: Health Systems and Nursing

Silvia Helena De Bortoli Cassiani, PhD, MSC, RN
Regional Advisor for Nursing, Pan American Health Organization

Bruna Moreno Dias, MSC, RN
Consultant at Pan American Health Organization
Health Systems and Services Department

Patricia Ingram-Martin, MS, RN
Chief Nursing Officer, Ministry of Health and Wellness of Jamaica

Casimiro Canha Cavaco Dias, MPH, MBA
Pan American Health Organization Advisor
Health Systems and Services for Jamaica, Bermuda, and the Cayman Islands

In 2020, the COVID-19 pandemic impacted services and health outcomes, particularly in marginalized populations, and highlighted the inextricable linkages between health, economy, environment, and social protection policies and mechanisms. The healthcare workforce has been hit hard by the pandemic, which exposed a chronic underinvestment. As health systems surged capacity, countries faced challenges in the human resources for health (HRH) on the front lines (Pan American Health Organization [PAHO], 2021).

Nurses and other healthcare professionals were and have been pivotal in the response, prevention, treatment, care, and rehabilitation of patients with COVID-19. Now it is time to advocate for more investments in the nursing workforce.

There are 8.4 million nursing personnel (30% of the nurses in the world) with a density of 83.4 nurses per 10,000 population in the region of the Americas. There are almost 10 times more nurses in the Americas than in the African region (World Health Organization [WHO], 2020). Nurses represent 56% of the total health workforce; 87% of the personnel are female and 13% male. Data informs that this region produces 81.2 nursing graduates per 100,000 population. This is the highest number in all regions of WHO (2020).

In October 2014, the PAHO and its member states adopted the Strategy for Universal Access to Health and Universal Health Coverage (PAHO, 2014). In 2016, the United Nations High-Level Commission on Health Employment and Economic Growth clearly conveyed that investing in the health workforce can accelerate progress across many of the sustainable development goals and can increase women's economic participation. Globally, 70% of workers in the health and social sectors are women (WHO, 2016).

> "Today we benefit from an ever-increasing evidence base for practice, production of nurse scientists, commitment to social responsibility, imperative to lead change in healthcare, and recognition that we are interdependent with other nations without restriction of borders. We care for the world and embrace our advocacy role to ensure that healthcare is a human right. The International Council of Nurses' (ICN) Code of Ethics for Nurses includes an explicit provision for nurses and global health (ICN, 2021). The American Nurses Association Code of Ethics for Nurses with Interpretive Statements (ANA, 2015) also underscores health as a universal right in Provision 8, which states, 'The nurse collaborates with other health professionals and the public to protect human rights, promote health diplomacy, and reduce health disparities.'"
>
> –Pamela F. Cipriano, PhD, RN, NEA-BC, FAAN
> President, International Council of Nurses
> Sadie Heath Cabaniss Professor and Dean, University of
> Virginia School of Nursing

In September 2017, PAHO approved the Strategy on Human Resources for Universal Health, intended to guide national policies on HRH. The lines of action of the strategy are: strengthen and consolidate governance and leadership in HRH; develop conditions and capacities to expand access to health and health coverage, with equity and quality; and partner with the education sector to respond to the needs of health systems in transformation toward universal health (PAHO, 2017). The documents reinforced that the shortage of HRH could compromise the achievement of universal health and, accordingly, the strengthening of the first level of care in health services.

Even before the pandemic, there were challenges such as leadership, stewardship, and management capacity to advance education, health, employment, and gender agendas; optimize return of current investments through adoption of required policy options; and generate massive investment and leverage them for outcomes, including job creation, gender, and youth empowerment. In 2020, it was recommended by WHO that national policy dialogues were conducted as one opportunity to enhance stakeholder input in policy development to reduce institutional barriers and leverage opportunities for changes and health reforms (Berman et al., 2019; Nabyonga-Orem et al., 2016).

The first country to conclude its policy dialogue was Uruguay. Uruguay has a shortage of registered nurses. There are two universities; however, it is difficult for this deficit to be reversed without national investments and policies. In 2021, the team appointed by the Ministry of Health generated forums with leaders to discuss the situation of national nursing shortages. The main conclusions were: equalize salaries in the public and private spheres; increase the number of nurses at the first level of care; decentralize nursing services and staff and encourage improved working conditions and salaries in the interior of the country; establish leadership positions; strengthen the role of nursing in health teams; create jobs that allow the implementation of public policies in education (school nurses), care to immigrants, and occupational health; and integrate nursing graduates into management teams at all management levels (Comisión Nacional de Enfermería & Organización Panamericana de la Salud, 2022).

Jamaica is another country that has conducted activities to develop the National Strategic Direction of Nursing and Midwifery. Currently, the Ministry of Health and Wellness is developing the Strategic Plan for Nursing and Midwifery (SPNM) in Jamaica through a broad and participative process. This plan will address the strategic priorities of jobs, education, practice, and leadership, mirroring the strategic priorities of the WHO *Global Strategic Directions for Nursing and Midwifery 2021–2025* (2021). The SPNM is being developed by four technical working groups and a steering committee of nursing and midwifery experts in both private and public sectors, supported by PAHO and the University of West Indies School of Nursing as the PAHO/WHO Collaborating Center. The Strategic Plan will guide the main reforms in Jamaica in the next five years for strengthening nursing and midwifery toward universal health.

Although the region of the Americas has made some progress in HRH, inequities persist in the availability, distribution, and quality of the nursing workforce. Precarious working conditions, low productivity, and poor performance are some of the challenges that countries are facing. In the next years, analysis of the workforce among the countries should be combined with labor market, gender, and fiscal space analyses to guide the development of policy options, strategies, and financing reforms. Further investments in workforce capacity will be essential to ensure preparedness for public health emergencies, such as COVID-19.

References

American Nurses Association. (2015). *Code of ethics for nurses with interpretive statements*. Author. https://www.nursingworld.org/coe-view-only

Berman, P., Azhar, A., & Osborn, E. J. (2019). Towards universal health coverage: Governance and organisational change in ministries of health. *BMJ Global Health*, 4(5), e001735. https://doi.org/10.1136/bmjgh-2019-001735

Comisión Nacional de Enfermería & Organización Panamericana de la Salud. (2022). *Nursing policy dialogue – Uruguay 2021*. Montevideo.

International Council of Nurses. (2021). *The ICN code of ethics for nurses, revised 2021*. https://www.icn.ch/system/files/2021-10/ICN_Code-of-Ethics_EN_Web_0.pdf

Nabyonga-Orem, J., Dovlo, D., Kwamie, A., Nadege, A., Guangya, W., & Kirigia, J. M. (2016). Policy dialogue to improve health outcomes in low income countries: What are the issues and way forward? *BMC Health Services Research, 16*(S4), 217. https://doi. org/10.1186/s12913-016-1450-2

Pan American Health Organization. (2014). *Strategy for universal access to health and universal health coverage.* https://iris.paho.org/handle/10665.2/28276

Pan American Health Organization. (2017). *Strategy on human resources for universal access to health and universal health coverage.* https://www.paho.org/en/documents/strategy-human-resources-universal-access-health-and-universal-health-coverage-csp2910

Pan American Health Organization. (2021). *CD59/11 – Strategy for building resilient health systems and post COVID-19 pandemic recovery to sustain and protect public health gains.* https://www.paho.org/en/documents/cd5911-strategy-building-resilient-health-systems-and-post-covid-19-pandemic-recovery

World Health Organization. (2016). *High-level commission on health employment and economic growth: Report of the expert group.* https://apps.who.int/iris/handle/10665/250040

World Health Organization. (2020). *State of the world's nursing report – 2020.* https://www. who.int/publications/i/item/9789240003279

World Health Organization. (2021). *Global Strategic Directions for Nursing and Midwifery 2021–2025.* https://www.who.int/publications/i/item/9789240033863

Addressing the Worldwide Nursing Workforce Shortage: "There's no justice . . . just us"

Dame Anne Marie Rafferty, DPhil (Oxon), FAAN, FRCN
Professor of Health & Nursing Policy, King's College London

Natalie Sanford, MSN, RN
PhD candidate, King's College London

The cruel and illegal war in Ukraine and author Terry Pratchett's immortal words, "there's no justice . . . just us," ring tragically true (2013, p. 86). The tangible consequences of the war, including flattened cities, destroyed infrastructure, collapsed health services, and civilian atrocities, will leave scars that will take decades to heal for the Ukrainian people, refugees, and the world. Rising costs of living and soaring energy prices are only the beginning of the devastating ripple effects of the war, both of which disproportionately impact the poor. This, in addition to the aftermath of an unprecedented global pandemic, expose with forensic cruelty how the most disadvantaged are societally abandoned and thus fare worse. This is particularly the case for marginalized communities, such as people with disabilities, the LGBTQ community, the BIPOC community, women, those of low socioeconomic status, and children. Nursing grew out of a reform movement targeted to alleviate poverty in the 19th century (Nelson & Rafferty, 2010). This was what animated Florence Nightingale and her allies, hence her interest in building health literacy through her famous "Notes on Nursing," district and community nursing as "The Star of Bethlehem," and the hospital as a place that should do the sick no harm. Nightingale understood disadvantage deeply and saw nursing as the most practical intervention to help resolve it.

Nurses work in a huge range of settings, armed with a panoply of skills and talents. Throughout the COVID-19 pandemic, these skills have been at the fore and have been the force that has saved many patients' lives. COVID-19, especially in its early days, was and is nursing work. Recently at a mental health conference, we had the glorious privilege of meeting face to face to celebrate advances and innovations sprung from locals in practice. There were nurses developing new risk assessment and safety measures for patients in forensic service in the health and justice services, piloting safeguarding techniques for looking after children in school, devising care packages for Ukrainian refugees centered around trauma-informed care, expanding offerings for women as victims of domestic abuse due to the increases in domestic violence during the pandemic, and increasing initiatives for the recruitment of refugee nurses themselves. The conference showcased the incredible work of talented nurses, working at the margins of society and finding ingenious ways to make a difference.

It is a tragic truism that the world is short of nurses to close the gap between the rich and the poor, and this gap is itself a moving target. The State of the World's Nursing Report (World Health Organization [WHO], 2020) estimated a 6 million shortfall out of 28 million in nursing numbers. These numbers are staggering and are also likely a huge underestimate. Our workforce planning centers mainly on supply rather than demand and does not account for the impact of the burdens of the pandemic on nurse mental health, retention, and retirement. The maldistribution of nurse provision in health economies mirrors inequalities between high- and low-income countries, such that there is a ten-fold decrease in the nurse-to-patient ratio between the US and some sub-Saharan countries (WHO, 2022).

There are severe consequences of the nursing shortage for the strength of health systems globally. The UN cannot meet its sustainable development goals (SDGs) in any domain without nurses. Nurses work in many settings, and a systemic approach to inequity is needed. Only an estimated 20% of health is driven by health services, with the majority being the product of education, housing, transport, climate, and sustainable environments—in short, the remaining SDGs (Magnan, 2017). Nurses save lives and are associated with increased quality of care, decreased patient mortality, decreased healthcare spending, and improved outcomes. Furthermore, inadequate staffing undermines patient confidence in health services. Hence, governments need to pay attention to nurses, with whom significant political capital is invested by the public.

What can we do to steward the future? Taking a leaf from the Nightingale playbook, we need to intervene at every level of the system—globally, nationally, and locally. The Nursing Now campaign has mobilized the power of the nursing voice. Now it needs to be organized and orchestrated with clear messaging on ending the nursing shortage and investing in nurse education and human capital. The triple impact of doing so will deliver on gender, employment, and educational outcomes for society, benefiting governments, patients, and population health (All-Party Parliamentary Group on Global Health, 2016). We must build on the UN Commission on Employment and Economy as well the WHO Assembly Resolution on Nursing and Midwifery (WHO, 2021), using these recommendations as our calling card to hold governments to account and translate these into tangible strategic goals to influence policy at every opportunity: the G7, G20, World Economic Summit, European Commission, and WHO and UN assemblies. Indeed, we need to infiltrate every multilateral venue where health is discussed and insist on a seat at the table, to talk not only to health ministers but education and finance ministers too. But most of all, this needs careful choreography and coordination, political craftsmanship, and leadership on a scale as never before.

Using all the available networks we have, we must activate our influence to steward the nursing workforce, speak with one voice, and stem the tide of growing health inequity while we still can. This approach has been taken before with similarly detrimental and global issues, such as climate change. Climate change looked like an insurmountable problem, but slowly it has been accepted that we can change its course, and governments now take responsibility for doing so. We need something similar for the nursing and health workforce. Like climate change, this is a catastrophe that is already happening. We need a Paris Treaty to set targets for policy goals and sanctions for nations who infringe on these targets. Perhaps a new legal framework/instrument of health governance will be needed. We, as healthcare professionals, must champion this cause; as Terry Pratchett decreed: "there is no justice . . . just us!"

References

All-Party Parliamentary Group on Global Health. (2016, October). *Triple impact – How developing nursing will improve health, promote gender equality and support economic growth.* https://ccoms.esenfc.pt/pub/DIGITAL%20APPG%20Triple%20Impact.pdf

Magnan, S. (2017). Social determinants of health 101 for health care: Five plus five. *NAM Perspectives.* [Discussion Paper, National Academy of Medicine]. https://doi.org/10.31478/201710c

Nelson, S., & Rafferty, A. M. (Eds.). (2010). *Notes on Nightingale: The influence and legacy of a nursing icon.* Cornell University Press.

Pratchett, T. (2013). *Mort.* Gollancz.

World Health Organization. (2020). *State of the world's nursing report.* https://www.who.int/publications/i/item/9789240003279

World Health Organization. (2021). *Global strategic directions for nursing and midwifery 2021–2025.* https://www.who.int/publications/i/item/9789240033863

World Health Organization. (2022). Global Health Workforce Statistics. https://www.who.int/data/gho/data/themes/topics/health-workforce

Global Stewardship: Reimagining the Adage "Think Global, Act Local" in the Post-Pandemic World—Every Nurse's Business

Jill White, PhD, MEd, MHPol, RN, AM, RM
Professor Emerita of the Susan Wakil School of Nursing and Midwifery
University of Sydney

There is not very much that I am grateful to the Coca-Cola Company for: not sugary drinks that increase childhood obesity, not bottled water adding to household costs and to plastic in landfill and oceans. I am grateful, however, that the company resurrected a near forgotten Scottish saying, "Think global, act local." First attributed to Patrick Geddes in the early 1900s in relation to the importance of local character in town planning, it was co-opted by Coca-Cola in the late 1990s as a focus for its marketing strategy, now adopted by the World Health Organization (WHO).

> *"Fundamental to nursing are concepts of equity, access, and social justice. These have local and global antecedents and impacts. Actions nurses choose to take are reflective of our professional identity and sense of social responsibility. It is about consciousness and professional conscience.*
> *'Think global, act local' is something every nurse can do. 'Act global, think local' is what our global nursing organizations are tasked to do with us and for us."*
>
> –Jill White, PhD, MEd, MHPol, RN, AM, RM
> Professor Emerita of the Susan Wakil School of Nursing and Midwifery, University of Sydney

In this strange post-pandemic world where it has been demonstrated beyond doubt that health and illness lines on a map have little meaning, how might "Think global, act local" help nurses become more active contributors to both local and global health-related concerns and the layers of decision-making and influence that lie between?

Every nursing encounter is influenced by decisions made beyond the nurse-patient dyad: staffing allocations/ratios, the resources available for care, the state of the facilities in which care takes place, the remuneration for nursing services, the out-of-pocket costs for patients and their families, regulation of scope of practice, etc. These decisions are, in turn, influenced at state and national levels by vigorously contested priorities for turf protection and scarce financial resources, argued by lobbyists, ministers of health, and ministers of finance and treasury. In turn, national decisions are influenced by current and predicted global events, such as pandemics, oil prices, and geopolitical stability. The COVID-19 pandemic displayed this layered interconnection vividly—global institutions like WHO provided evidence and technical advice as it became available; governments and Big Pharma made deals about price, availability, and purchase of vaccines; governments made choices about release of national stocks of personal protective equipment and ventilators and made choices related to compulsory vaccination of health workers, border closures, and quarantine restrictions and facilities. These high-level decisions rippled right to the bedside and changed the day-to-day working lives of nurses and their interactions with their patients and communities in every country.

Nurses can accept this buffeting as beyond their control, or they can, in seeing the interconnections, participate at a local level, while simultaneously understanding the impacts at a global level and the levels in between. I like to think of this as being able to hold a close-up patient-focused view (seeing near) whilst also being able to appreciate the long-distance view (seeing far) and their interconnection. The key to participation is understanding the politics of policymaking. To be successful in policy influence at any level, one must have both the evidence and the story of the impact of the problem to be solved. Nurses often think that if they can present this evidence to policymakers with a compelling story, then surely action would be taken. Not so.

One must also be acutely aware of and attuned to the context of the proposed change (budgets, world events, elections, etc.). One must understand the policy process and that engagement at the stages of problem definition and solution proposing is critical, because by the time a policy gets to a consultation table, it is largely complete. Finally, one must understand the stakeholders—who are the actors, what are their interests, and who are the powerful lobby groups who might be negatively affected (Buse et al., 2012)? If one uses this lens of analysis on policy and change whether at the unit level, community level, national level, or global level, the likelihood of having effective influence is greatly enhanced.

Nurses know the full gamut of what it takes to provide care under the most extraordinary circumstances. This cumulative story must be part of the rebuilding of health services. The pandemic has shown the cracks in the current health systems at all levels. As Leonard Cohen once prophetically said of the cracks in things, "that's where the light gets in," and as health systems are reformed, nursing voices must be heard (1992).

This interconnectivity from local to global and the political policy process that underpins it have rarely been part of the nursing curriculum. Understanding the broader arena of practice, given its impact on practice possibilities, must surely be part of the learning of the nurse. Take the example of climate change: Many nurses, while seeing climate change as real and threatening, do not see a connection between their work as a nurse and climate change. Yet the scenarios of fires and floods are a direct consequence of climate change in Australia. Predictions of warming will also alter food production and people's ability to deal with temperature changes, with the elderly and the already marginalized groups at greatest risk.

Practice will be impacted, and this makes it a nursing matter. So, what can nurses do about it? We can work at every level of influence from the bedside to the boardroom to the United Nations. In many countries there are the beginnings of action, such as that at King Edward in Perth, Australia, where nurses are deeply engaged in a project to reduce the waste of single-use plastics to prevent the massive hospital waste that now goes into landfills and finds its way into the oceans. Nurses are lobbying hospital boards to move to renewable energy sources such as solar power. Nurses are joining protests about the extension of gas-fired power stations and the further expansion of coal mining. These projects are recognized by nurses as not only dislocating families from otherwise productive farming land, with mental health consequences, but also adding to the air pollution—local and global effects. Nurses are active participants in organizations such as the Climate and Health Alliance (https://www.caha.org.au/), which in turn link to global organizations such as Global Green and Healthy Hospitals (https://www.greenhospitals.net/).

These stories of concrete actions are taken up at the national level through national nursing organizations (NNO) to our global nursing organizations, such as the International Council of Nurses, Sigma, and the office of the Global Chief Nurse at WHO. They then work in two directions, producing evidence-based position papers to come back to NNOs and making links at the global level with like-minded organizations for greater influence.

There is nothing nurses do that does not have consequences ultimately for their patients, the community, the country, and the planet: waste reduction at home or at work; active collaboration in evidence-informed and locally applied practice; or voting knowledgeably and consciously, considering policies of health, education, women's issues such as domestic violence, family planning, and mental health. We can make a difference. That is global stewardship.

References

Buse, K., Mays, N., & Walt, G. (2012). *Making health policy* (2nd ed). Open University Press.

Cohen, L. (1992). Anthem [Song]. *The Future* [Album]. Columbia Records.

Thirty3

Music & Lyrics Written by Tad Worku

Tad Worku is a songwriter, singer, speaker, and nurse practitioner. His music is available via most music streaming services. You can find out more at tadworku.com.

Back Story: I wrote this song after having a conversation with an 83-year-old woman in the ED who had terminal cancer and a few weeks left to live. After developing rapport I asked her, "What season of life would you live over again if you could?" She answered, "This one." I was surprised and asked her why. She said that she was at peace, was surrounded by the people she loved, and had faith. That conversation impacted me and reminded me that every situation and season of life has something meaningful in it. Even in her final season of life, she still found meaning.

V1
Seven years, no you're not that old
Wake up to a brand new day, every day
Count the minutes oh they move so slow

Peace to find, can be hard at 29
Throw a rock at 30, just a step away
All downhill at least that's what they say

PRE-CHORUS
But do you believe them
Or does every season in life have a reason a morsel to glean
To tell myself at 18

V2
Life won't end, no not at 42
Learning from the journey that you're walking through
Hurry up cause time won't wait for you

64, tell me what your living for
Is life about the moments that you wish you had
Does the love around you make you glad?

CHORUS
And do you believe them
Or does every season in life have a reason a morsel to glean
To tell myself at 16

V3
83, She smiled and looked at me
Said you're just a baby at 32
the best of life is still in front of you

CHORUS
She said don't stop believing
That every seasons in life has a reason a morsel to glean
She said count your blessings not time
Live to love and you'll find you will be
Ready for 33

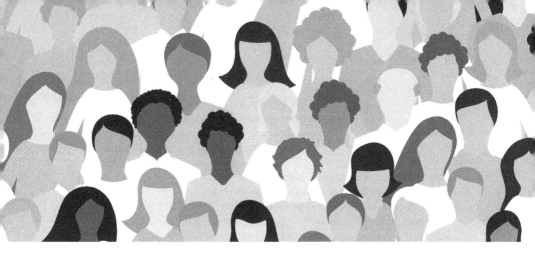

10 Nursing's Voice in Leading Change

In This Chapter

- Unmute Us: The Power of Diverse Voices in Nursing and Leadership

- Finding Our Voice of Advocacy

- Voice of Nursing From the Front Lines

- Pandemic School Nursing—Another Front Line

- Nurses You Should Know: Inclusive Storytelling Designed to Expand the Nursing Narrative

- The Voice of Advocacy: If Not You, Then Who?

Since the inception of the profession, nurses have been an ever-present force in healthcare and the community. Our presence has expanded to occupy spaces that our nursing predecessors may have never imagined, and thus, our voices have grown louder and stronger. The nurse's voice can be heard in Congress leading policy change, on farms cultivating nutritious crops for the community, in government intelligence agencies on top secret missions, in C-suites making executive-level decisions, and at protests marching for social justice. The nurse's voice is everywhere! The nurse's voice is awe-inspiring in its ability to motivate change, and we cannot afford to lower our voices one single decibel. The right to quality, consistent healthcare is at stake, especially for people of color and those who live in poverty, and the voice of nursing is poised to lead change. We must come together collectively to unite with a zealous voice to advocate for change— to demand health equity!

Consider the following questions as you read the essays about how the nurse's voice can lead to change in health equity:

- In what ways can nurses go beyond patient and client care to encourage health equity?

- List unique spaces or occupations in which you have seen nurses lead.

- What are examples of how nurses in your community fight for health equity?

- In what ways are nurses equipped to lead the change for health equity?

- How can you use your voice to lead the change for health equity?

Unmute Us: The Power of Diverse Voices in Nursing and Leadership

Paule Valery Joseph, PhD, MS, FNP-BC, CRNP, FAAN
Lasker Clinical Research Scholar
National Institute on Alcohol Abuse and Alcoholism
National Institutes of Health

Imagine a world in healthcare where the voices of nurses from diverse backgrounds, from the bedside to the boardroom, are heard when promoting change, diversity, and health equity. Despite significant advances in science and public health during the past few decades, healthcare disparities exist throughout the United States. The COVID-19 pandemic highlighted the deep inequalities in the US health system. Communities of color are more likely than whites to experience pervasive disparities that worsen health outcomes. Nurses are uniquely positioned to see how social injustice destroys patients' and communities' health and welfare and to act towards achieving health equity. Nursing is the nation's largest healthcare profession, often ranked the most trusted profession, with over 4 million registered nurses nationwide and the primary providers of hospital patient care (American Association of Colleges of Nursing, 2022). As patient advocates and stewards of health, our nursing voices have never been more critical in achieving health equity. Nursing students and nurses at all levels must be actively involved and engaged in enacting change in the healthcare system to achieve health equity. Our voices as nurses have the power to impact positive changes in nursing practice and health equity to improve patient care.

"When nurses speak with one voice that health equity work is fundamentally quality care work, in both policy and practice, a mighty blow will be struck to structural racism. When organizations understand the population being served and reflect the population being served, the old structure will begin to crumble. Value-based care is about metrics, structure, and intentionality—what and how are you trying to achieve. Nurses, let's be intentional."

–Rita Wray, MBA, RN, BC, FAAN
Founder & Chief Executive Officer, Wray Enterprises, Inc.

Health equity is social justice. Nursing has been built on social justice and community health advocacy. Nurses must speak up about racial disparities by educating themselves and others on how systemic racism impacts health outcomes and healthcare delivery. Many professional nursing organizations have condemned racism as a public health issue in the last two years. Yet, this is not enough, as it is imperative that all nurses use their voices to address the racism within the nursing profession, as most nurses of color report workplace racism (American Nurses Association [ANA], 2022). As nurses, we must acknowledge areas where we, our departments, or our organizations may be treating patients and colleagues unequally or inequitably. As leaders for equity, we must examine, unpack, and mitigate our own biases and dismantle the policies and structures that hold inequity in place. Our success in creating organizations, schools, and communities where everyone has access to the opportunities they need to thrive depends on our willingness to confront the history and the impact of systemic racism.

As a profession, we cannot stay silent; remaining silent about racial injustices has alarming consequences and perpetuates inequalities. According to the Code of Ethics for Nurses (ANA, 2015), we must advance health and human rights and reduce disparities. Despite our ethical mandate, many nurses are not prepared for or willing to have conversations related to social justice. We know that until we dismantle structural racism and reimagine a society premised upon racial, social, economic, gender, and environmental justice, our patients will not be able to achieve and maintain the optimal health we wish for them. We have unique roles to play in the movement for racial justice and must act now. Nurses are uniquely positioned to advocate for antiracism policies throughout the healthcare system. Our profession is responsible for being antiracist rather than "not racist."

Nurses need to fulfill the tenets dictated by our nursing profession to serve and provide optimal care for the betterment of human health and human lives regardless of race, ethnicity, or socioeconomic constructs. Nurses must use their voices to highlight how, for many patients and nurses of color like me, it goes beyond encountering a glass ceiling but instead hitting a concrete wall. We must be committed to change, but it is critical that in this process of creating the change, we are thoughtful as a profession not to call on nurses and nurse faculty of color disproportionately to serve on committees—perpetuating more disparities with the so-called "Black tax." As we move forward, we must also be committed to addressing racism by critically looking at the past and the present and acknowledging the many contributions and experiences of nurses of color who are often omitted or silenced. Our voices can challenge the systems and policies that have led to generations of injustices and racial and ethnic health inequities.

Although the COVID-19 pandemic highlighted the indispensable value of nursing across the spectrum of healthcare and science, the voices of nurses often remain in the background, exerting little influence on health policy, patient care, and research, especially representation of nurses from historically excluded groups. Nurses are rarely involved in informing policy and are often underrepresented on many boards and healthcare task forces (Walton et al., 2015). Although now we have more nurses in legislative roles, it is not enough. We need more nurses of diverse backgrounds serving on private, local, state, and federal task forces that draft policy and legislation. In addition, we need to provide opportunities for nursing students and nurses working at the bedside to be engaged in health leadership early. For example, in the era of increased misinformation, nurses can use their voices to be at the forefront of stopping the spread of misinformation. We have the skills and are uniquely positioned to inform the public about important issues, complex problems, and discoveries. The accomplishments and failures learned in how to communicate science during COVID-19 have valuable lessons for the profession. We need to advocate for more nurses in science journalism and science communication to be included in undergraduate and graduate programs. Nurses use their voices to ensure patients' access to care through advocacy and shape public policy.

In conclusion, having nurses committed to social justice and actively engaged in health policy leadership ensures the inclusion of diverse voices to impact patients' health and health outcomes. Diversity in boards and leadership positions brings a unique understanding of systemic issues that affect health outcomes. Including nurses can help organizations improve racial health disparities and employee and patient experiences. A commitment to social justice and advocacy is a commitment to improving patient outcomes and improving health equity.

Disclaimer: This material should not be interpreted as representing the viewpoint of the US Department of Health and Human Services, the National Institutes of Health, or the National Institute on Alcohol Abuse and Alcoholism.

References

American Association of Colleges of Nursing. (2022). *Nursing fact sheet.* https://www.aacnnursing.org/News-Information/Fact-Sheets/Nursing-Fact-Sheet

American Nurses Association. (2015). *Code of ethics for nurses with interpretive statements.* Author. https://www.nursingworld.org/coe-view-only

American Nurses Association. (2022). *New survey data: Racism within the nursing profession is a substantial problem.* https://www.nursingworld.org/news/news-releases/2021/new-survey-data-racism-in-nursing/

Walton, A., Lake, D., Mullinix, C., Allen, D., & Mooney, K. (2015). Enabling nurses to lead change: The orientation experiences of nurses to boards. *Nursing Outlook, 63*(2), 110–116. https://doi.org/10.1016/j.outlook.2014.12.015

Finding Our Voice of Advocacy

Deborah T. Zimmermann, DNP, RN, NEA-BC, FAAN
Chief Executive Officer, DAISY Foundation
President, American Organization for Nursing Leadership

By 2030, 20% of US citizens will be over age 65, and of those, 85% are predicted to be afflicted with at least one chronic illness requiring nursing care (Fong, 2019). Populations with lower incomes are generally associated with higher rates of morbidity and mortality (Berchick et al., 2018), and the impact of the COVID-19 pandemic significantly affected disadvantaged populations. The elderly, populations living in poverty, and Black and Latinx people experienced disproportionately higher rates of hospitalization and deaths from COVID-19 (Berchick et al., 2018; Getachew et al., 2020). Almost 50% of the Latinx and Black population reported financial challenges and job losses (Parker et al., 2020), which glaringly exposed racial and social disparities.

> *"For some, the link between nursing and policy may not seem obvious, but the reality is that nurses transform evidence into action every day by using their voice to advocate for patient needs. This voice makes nurses particularly well-suited to influence policies that lead to more equitable health outcomes."*
>
> –Alison K. Hernandez, PhD, RN-BC
> Policy Advisor, Washington, DC

Nursing Success in Underserved Areas

In 2009, the American Academy of Nursing began recognizing innovative, nurse-led programs that reduced cost, improved care, and enhanced patient satisfaction as Edge Runners (American Academy of Nurses, n.d.; Ford-Roegner & Parry, 2009). A few years later, the American Academy of Ambulatory Care Nursing (2017) published a paper calling for registered nurses to transform healthcare from a medical model to a team-based system with a focus on disease prevention, health promotion, and cost containment. In communities across the US, programs led by nurses and directed at specific disadvantaged populations such as single first-time parents, adults with chronic illness, seniors, and children emerged.

Consistently, these small and cost-effective programs demonstrated sustained reductions in hospital readmissions, inpatient complications, mortality rates, and healthcare costs while improving patient access, addressing social disparities, and embracing patient-centered approaches to care (Kitzman, et al., 2019; Martsolf et al., 2016; Peter et al., 2011; Raftery et al., 2005). A survey of Edge Runners found that nurse-led programs provided social support, holistic-culturally sensitive care, and were built on trust (Mason et al., 2018).

Why, then, have these successful and largely local programs not been embraced as national models and received funding or support from accrediting bodies for expansion? One answer may be that the US health system is founded on a problem-oriented medical model. Healthcare focuses on cure rather than health (Martsolf et al., 2016). Engaging and persuading payors, the Centers for Medicare and Medicaid Services, and accrediting agencies like the Joint Commission can be daunting endeavors. Nurses may feel intimidated by the process or lacking in expertise.

Another explanation for the modest growth in nurse-led programs may lie within the profession itself. The American Nurses Association Barriers to Registered Nurse Scope of Practice Professional Issues Panel suggested the limitation of nursing's influence is in part self-inflicted, and the responsibility to effect change rests with us (Williams et al., 2016). We have not traditionally used our power as the largest healthcare profession or our voice to influence national committees on healthcare strategy. The panel suggested that as professionals, we have the responsibility to determine and control our scope of practice; as advocates, we have a responsibility to influence the care environment; as innovators, we promote and serve as agents of change; and lastly, we are collaborators, partners, and leaders of healthcare (Williams et al., 2016). The panel specifically called for us to collaborate with accrediting bodies, to become strategists, and not accept barriers as "blockades to action" (Williams et al., 2016, p. 11). Finally, they contend it is our responsibility to overcome these constraints and show the nation a better way to better health.

Tipping Point for Change

For the 20th consecutive year, nurses were rated the most trusted and ethical profession (Gallup, 2022). Nurse-led innovations like those mentioned here have improved clinical outcomes, expanded access to care, broken down racial barriers, and incorporated patient-centered approaches to care. Nurses were instrumental in developing community, state, and national COVID-19 responses to the pandemic. There is now greater public awareness of the need for sustainable cultures of health, the elimination of social disparities, and the creation of robust environments for clinician well-being.

Your voice, your knowledge, and your advocacy are vital. Begin the journey of advocating for change by meeting with a finance colleague in your organization. Share data and influence using your knowledge. As nurses, we are conveners, educators, advocates, and innovators. The disruption caused by the pandemic provides a great window of opportunity.

Convene the team that will advocate for expanded coverage and payment of nurse-led programs. Together:

- Develop an agenda that informs the nursing community, healthcare professionals, and political stakeholders of the value and cost-effectiveness of nurse-led programs.

- Partner with regulatory agencies, legislators, and payors to remove barriers for nurses to practice at their full scope of licensure. Invite them to join you at the table; they too will benefit from the relationship.

Conclusion

A community is only as healthy as its most disadvantaged populations. Commit to advancing the agenda of the American Academy of Nursing and the National Academy of Medicine (American Academy of Nurses, n.d.; National Academies of Sciences, Engineering, and Medicine, 2021) by advocating for the expansion of nurse-led innovations into health policy and practice. We must all assume broader and more formal roles in healthcare redesign.

References

American Academy of Ambulatory Care Nursing. (2017). *American Academy of Ambulatory Care Nursing position paper: The role of the registered nurse in ambulatory care.* https://www.aaacn.org/sites/default/files/documents/RNRolePositionPaper.pdf

American Academy of Nurses. (n.d.). *Edge runners.* https://www.aannet.org/initiatives/edge-runners

Berchick, E. R., Hood, E., & Barnett, J. C. (2018). *Health insurance coverage in the United States: 2017.* https://www.census.gov/content/dam/Census/library/publications/2018/demo/p60-264.pdf

Fong, J. H. (2019). Disability incidence and functional decline among older adults with major chronic diseases. *BMC Geriatrics, 19*(1), 323. https://doi.org/10.1186/s12877-019-1348-z

Ford-Roegner, M., & Parry, L. (2009). Nurse edge runners – The hallmark of the Raise the Voice campaign. *Nursing Outlook, 57*(5), 296–297.

Gallup. (2022, January 21). *Military brass, judges among professions at new image lows.* https://news.gallup.com/poll/388649/military-brass-judges-among-professions-new-image-lows.aspx

Getachew, Y., Zephyrin, L., Abrams, M. K., Shah, A., Lewis, C., & Doty, M. M. (2020, September 10). *Beyond the case count: The widespread disparities of COVID-19 in the United States.* Commonwealth Fund. https://www.commonwealthfund.org/sites/default/files/2020-09/Getachew_beyond_case_count_COVID_disparities_sb_v2.pdf

Kitzman, H., Olds, D. L., Knudtson, M. D., Cole, R., Anson, E., Smith, J. A., Fishbein, D., DiClemente, R., Wingood, G., Caliendo, A. M., Hopfer, C., Miller, T., & Conti, G. (2019). Prenatal and infancy nurse home visiting and 18-year outcomes of a randomized trial. *Pediatrics, 144*(6), e20183876. https://doi.org/10.1542/peds.2018-3876

Martsolf, G. R., Gordon, T., Warren May, L., Mason, D., Sullivan, C., & Villarruel, A. (2016). Innovative nursing care models and culture of health: Early evidence. *Nursing Outlook, 64*(4), 367–376. https://doi.org/10.1016/j.outlook.2016.02.009

Mason, D. J., Martsolf, G. R., Sloan, J., Villarruel, A., & Sullivan, C. (2018). Making health a shared value: Lessons from nurse-designed models of care. *Nursing Outlook, 67*(3), 213–222. https://doi.org/10.1016/j.outlook.2018.12.024

National Academies of Sciences, Engineering, and Medicine. (2021). *The future of nursing 2020–2030: Charting a path to achieve health equity.* The National Academies Press. https://nam.edu/publications/the-future-of-nursing-2020-2030

Parker, K., Minkin, R., & Bennett, J. (2020). *Economic fallout from COVID-19 continues to hit lower-income Americans the hardest.* Pew Research Center. https://www.pewsocialtrends.org/2020/09/24/economic-fallout-from-covid-19-continues-to-hit-lower-income-americans-the-hardest/

Peter, S., Chaney, G., Zappia, T., Van Veldhuisen, C., Pereira, S., & Santamaria, N. (2011). Care coordination for children with complex care needs. *Journal for Specialists in Pediatric Nursing, 16*(4), 305–312. https://doi.org/10.1111/j.1744-6155.2011.00303.x

Raftery, J. P., Yao, G. L., Murchie, P., Campbell, N. C., & Ritchie, D. (2005). Cost-effectiveness of nurse led secondary prevention clinics for coronary heart disease in primary care: Follow up of a randomized controlled trial. *British Medical Journal, 330*(7439), 707. https://doi.org/10.1136/bmj.38342.665417.8F

Williams, T. E., Baker, K., Evans, L., Lucatorto, M. A., Moss, E., O'Sullivan, A., Seifert, P. C., Siek, T., Thomas, T. W., & Zittel, B. (2016). Registered nurses as professionals, advocates, innovators, and collaborative leaders: Executive summary. *Online Journal of Issues in Nursing, 21*(3), 5. https://doi.org/10.3912/OJIN.Vol21No03Man05

Voice of Nursing From the Front Lines

Nacole Riccaboni, MSN, APRN, AGAC-NP
Nursing Content Creator

Although the media and some practitioners might see nurses as mere laborers, we are far from simple task masters. The word *care* doesn't even explain how many physical and cerebral checks and balances are involved in a single nurse performing one task. We are the eyes and ears of our community, especially for those underserved who might not be in a position to advocate for themselves. We are on the front lines as experts, and people trust us with their care. We care deeply about being entrusted with the overall health and well-being of individuals, families, and communities, especially those where disparities run deep. Being on the front lines gives us expertise in determining realistic expectations, available resources, and process improvements. The term *front line* has had much attention lately, but I do not think many individuals understand the power of that station, nurses included.

Serving as both the brain and the heart of the healthcare system, we must be compelled to use our voices to ensure the needs of our communities. Nurses assess, implement, and evaluate all aspects of healthcare distribution. We interact with individuals and move within this machine called healthcare. We see and operate the gauges, gears, pullies, and levers. We are the switches, relays, and electrical wiring that keep this entire process functioning. As nurses, we see the barriers and opportunities to improve all processes and protocols. Our impact can't be denied, and our voices must be listened to, accepted, appreciated, and valued.

Sadly, however, our input is often not weighed on the same level as those in more senior-level leadership positions. This aspect should not stop nurses from stepping forward and leading change. The change will not occur passively though. Change is an active and ongoing process that must include all nurses banding together. The role of change-maker is filled with grit and requires effort. We have that!

I am a nurse practitioner, and just a few years ago I was a critical care bedside nurse. I am not that far removed from the bedside now, but I expect that those on the front lines let me know when my expectations and goals are not suitable. Those distanced from the bedside must understand that they have a limited bird's-eye view. Frontline nurses are crucial in ensuring all processes are feasible, safe, appropriate, and positive. Nurses' input should not be a nicety or an option but rather a requirement. The nurse's voice should be the focus or central point of whether a proposal will work on a larger scale.

Nurses should be present on committees, leadership bodies, councils, and boards. They should be the individuals who are conduits to leadership in understanding what care involves, what the people need. Although each organization has its own set of goals, nurses can determine if those goals are feasible and appropriate, ensuring the proposed efforts will either positively or negatively impact patient care. You are a nurse filled with so much knowledge and talent, organizations and community groups would love to work with you. Nurses' unique experiences and exceptional problem-solving skills provide outlets and options other individuals can't tap into.

I have been present at leadership meetings with individuals who had many more credentials and longer resumes than I have, yet I felt that in many cases I best understood the situation from the patient's perspective. Can it be done, given the current setting and resources? How will this affect the patient and family? An idea is great, but it is doomed to fail if it is not feasible. Instead of simply focusing on your assignment or isolated concern, think about your overall job objectives, or what you believe needs changing, from a broader vision. Communicate your ideas and always provide the evidence and anecdotes to back them up.

Nurses do not need to be in formal leadership roles to have their voices heard. As nurses, we advocate all the time for our patients and for our institutions—as we have seen with the COVID-19 pandemic and the effects of our health system on people of color. We must be their voice. There is power in numbers. If multiple nurses are all facing the same issues, it is time your voices are heard. Speak to management, leadership, and community members for opportunities to enhance and amplify your voice, and always center your conversations on what is best for patients and families.

Do not make yourself small, your voice a whisper. Stand tall in knowing you are the key to patients and families getting exactly what they need to stay healthy and well. You are key to achieving health equity in this country. Let me say that again: *You* are the key to achieving health equity in this country . . . and in the world!

Pandemic School Nursing— Another Front Line

Robin Cogan, MEd, RN, NCSN, FAAN
Clinical Coordinator, School Nurse Specialty Program
Rutgers School of Nursing–Camden

The presence of a school nurse in every school was never more urgent than during the public health emergency of the COVID-19 pandemic. The essence of advocacy is influencing stakeholders or decision-makers through education, something in which school nurses, when given the opportunity, are experts. School nurses democratize access to healthcare for our most marginalized students and families. But 60% of schools in our country either have no school nurse (25%) or only a part-time nurse (35%), and 96,000 school nurses are tasked with caring for our nation's 56 million children (Willgerodt et al., 2018). There should be a school nurse in every building, every day, a concept supported by the American Academy of Pediatrics even prior to the pandemic (Holmes et al., 2016).

What we found during the early days of COVID-19 were community inequities of epic proportion—always present but never addressed. In urban school districts like Camden, New Jersey, where I have been a school nurse for the past 21 years, brick and mortar schools closed for more than a year beginning in March of 2020. We shifted to remote learning but found ways to address the complex social and health needs of students in innovative and collaborative ways.

Access to nutritious meals available for pickup and/or delivery was quickly established by the food services department of our school district. Connectivity became the holy grail of student success and was a primary focus at the beginning of the pandemic. Literal connectivity, and Wi-Fi access, which so many take for granted, were not available to the majority of our students. Donations and grants allowed my school district to provide students with devices and hotspots.

Pivoting is one word that will forever remind me of the pandemic. We pivoted so often that it felt like whiplash as we addressed each challenge head-on with creativity, rigor, compassion, and concern for the health, safety, and well-being of our school community. School nurses literally sewed masks in those early days because we had given all our personal protection equipment (PPE) to local acute care hospitals during the PPE shortages that plagued the early days of COVID-19. We created online health offices through Google Classroom and uploaded narrated stories to YouTube to read to our youngest students. We taught health lessons on Zoom and consulted with families of students with chronic health conditions by holding virtual school health office hours.

We had no road map for what we were about to encounter as en masse we started to reopen school buildings in the fall of 2021 after months of remote learning. The chorus we kept hearing was "we are building the plane as we are flying it"—a sentiment that did not instill confidence as we bravely entered school buildings with the most consequential charge, keeping students and staff safe through a global pandemic. School nurses became the next front line of COVID-19 without the resources or support needed to accomplish the untenable task of keeping other people's children safe.

I had experience amplifying the voice of school nurses through my blog, *The Relentless School Nurse* (Cogan, 2017). My blog has grown from several thousand readers in my first year in 2017 to over 300,000 readers to date. When the enormity of COVID-19 became apparent, I began to use my blog and social media presence to raise awareness about concerns that school nurses were facing.

Throughout the pandemic, I ran virtual support groups for school nurses through a grant from the Federal Emergency Management Agency and the Mental Health Association in New Jersey called New Jersey Hope and Healing. Each week school nurses from across the country shared their deepest concerns, challenges, and triumphs as we struggled through each phase of the pandemic. For more than 20 months, the group joined forces to support each other during the most consequential time in modern school nursing history.

The most common themes discussed during our more than 100 hours of weekly sessions were feeling disempowered, disrespected, silenced, and traumatized. Negative experiences with parents, who believed the school nurses were overreaching when it came to implementing COVID-19 guidelines, compounded the mounting stressors. Challenging school nurses' assessments by school staff through questioning decisions made to quarantine or send students home for COVID-19-like symptoms weighed heavily on the school nurses. Believing that our expertise in public health and communicable disease management was constantly under scrutiny and decisions were second-guessed led to school nurses feeling unheard and disbelieved. The untenable stressors of the front line of COVID-19 at school led to the early retirement or resignation of many school nurses (Nierenberg, 2021).

School nurses are the dedicated, licensed health professionals in a school community whose eyes and ears are an extension of both parents and staff. The role of the school nurse has morphed into the Chief Wellness Officer, even if that is not our official title! We are determined to use the collective strength and resolve we have gained through pandemic school nursing to address the many challenges of providing school health services to our nation's youth.

References

Cogan, R. (2017, July 6). The relentless school nurse: Will you be one too? *The Relentless School Nurse*. https://relentlessschoolnurse.com/2017/07/06/the-journey-begins/

Holmes, B. W., Sheetz, A., Allison, M., Ancona, R., Attisha, E., Beers, N., De Pinto, C., Gorski, P., Kjolhede, C., Lerner, M., Weiss-Harrison, A., & Young, T. (2016, June 1). Role of the school nurse in providing school health services. *American Academy of Pediatrics*. https://publications.aap.org/pediatrics/article/137/6/e20160852/52405/Role-of-the-School-Nurse-in-Providing-School

Nierenberg, A. (2021, November 17). School nurses feel like 'the enemy'. *The New York Times*. https://www.nytimes.com/2021/11/17/us/school-nurses-covid.html

Willgerodt, M. A., Brock, D. M., & Maughan, E. M. (2018). Public school nursing practice in the United States. *Journal of School Nursing, 34*(3), 232–244. https://doi.org/10.1177/1059840517752456

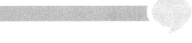

Nurses You Should Know: Inclusive Storytelling Designed to Expand the Nursing Narrative

Ravenne Aponte, BA, BSN, RN
PhD Student, University of Pennsylvania School of Nursing

Joanna Seltzer Uribe, EdD, MSN, RN
Johnson & Johnson Nurse Innovation Fellow

Documentation of healing practices has early roots in ancient Egypt that trace back nearly 5,000 years (Hunt, 2017). For centuries, people across the world have advocated, practiced healing traditions, and cared for patients with the goal of restoring health, preventing complications, and promoting comfort. Pre-professional nursing as a practice was shaped globally by various cultures and individuals who sought to address the health and social needs of the communities they served. This includes, but is not limited to, the Obregonian brotherhood of Madrid, Indigenous Mexican *parteras* (midwives) and *curanderos* (healers), Black midwives and herbalists, traditional Chinese nursing, and European sisterhoods (Hao et al., 2011). Despite the bravery and generations of acquired knowledge from such groups, including the first known nursing textbook by the Obregonian Catholic brotherhood in 1617, the dominant origin story of professional nursing begins with the strategic efforts of a single British nurse in the 1854 Crimean War, Florence Nightingale (Seltzer, 2021). While Nightingale, or "The Lady with the Lamp," is heralded as the founder of professional nursing, her vision also established who and what a nurse should look like that has endured for over a century. The 19th century design of modern nursing centered feminine, middle-class, anglophone, white, Christian women and established the profession by excluding those who did not fit the image of the Victorian-era "professional nurse."

Historians of nursing Sandra B. Lewenson and Eleanor Khron Horrman tell us, "History teaches us who we are" (Lewenson & Herrmann, 2008). Acknowledging the diversity of nursing's past and highlighting the experiences of nurses beyond Nightingale's model elicits an expanded origin story that seeks to include nurses of color, make their contributions to healthcare more widely known, and reshape our professional identity. History as a tool allows us to see the changes, different meanings, and experiences of nursing over time. Most importantly it serves as the foundation in which we can better understand and address contemporary nursing problems such as racism, workforce diversity, and health disparities. Nurses of color make up 20% of the nursing workforce, and subsequently their efforts and experiences have taken background to that of nursing's majority (Smiley et al., 2021). How might we amplify the stories of nurses of color who practice at the intersections of gender, race, class, and education levels?

Nursing informaticists and human-centered designers say, "Make the right thing the easy thing." Easy includes making "it"—the intervention, medication, antidote—accessible, affordable, findable, and feasible (Lengstorf, 2018). With that same philosophy, the Nurses You Should Know project was born. On Black History Month in 2021, an online learning platform that combined history and equity-centered community design was created to diversify the nursing narrative and show that all nurses belong in the profession (Creative Reaction Lab, 2022; Nurses You Should Know, 2022). Amidst the COVID-19 pandemic, where we transitioned to a nearly virtual world, the project delivered stories of past and present-day nurses of color directly to nurses' social media feeds, which "made the right thing the easy thing." These moments of micro-dosed digital learning brought the relevance of history to nurses' fingertips and served to narrow nursing's representation gap.

Transitioning the history of nursing to digestible bite-sized videos and blogs, the Nurses You Should Know project has highlighted over 100 nurse stories both past and present, from periods of Jim Crow segregation to nurse policymakers on Capitol Hill advocating for change in health policy in the 21st century. Black, Latinx, Asian, Pacific Islander, Native American, and Indigenous nurses share their journeys, challenges, wins, and hopes for the future of nursing. The platform serves to share our differences, backgrounds, education levels, and the various paths in which nurses of color have traveled. Most importantly, we look to the past to shine light on the nurses who blazed a trail for future nurses to follow. These nurses include but are not limited to:

- **Eva Carillo de Garcia:** Mexican American missionary nurse born in 1883 who would go on to advocate for Mexican American desegregation in Austin, Texas.

- **Maria Abastilla Beltran:** A public health nurse who immigrated from the Philippines to the United States in 1929 and established the Filipino Women's Club in Seattle.

- **Lula Owl Gloyne:** First Eastern Band Cherokee Indian registered nurse who advocated for the Bureau of Indian Affairs to build the first hospital for Cherokee people in 1937.

- **Colonel Lawrence Washington:** First male, and first Black male, in the Army Nurse Corps, who entered with the rank of 2nd lieutenant reserve officer in 1967 and served over 27 years as a psychiatric mental health nurse.

- **Sallie Tucker Allen:** Founder of the Association of Black Nursing Faculty and Tucker Publications, Inc., which sought to address the publishing gap of nurses of color in the late 1980s.

What these nurses show us is that despite the challenges, segregation, and limited opportunities in the first century of nursing, they continued to expand future opportunities for nurses of color. Generations of nurses of color, from the Civil War through today, fundamentally shaped the American nursing profession because when there was injustice in the profession or unequal delivery of care, they spoke up, organized, and advocated for the profession to course correct.

An example of this course correction is represented still today in the National Commission to Address Racism in Nursing. The commission—started in 2021 and led by the National Black Nurses Association, the National Coalition of Ethnic Minority Nurse Associations, the National Association of Hispanic Nurses, and the American Nurses Association—builds on decades of past efforts by nurses of color who identified and confronted racism within nursing to create a more inclusive and equitable future for nurses and patients.

So, when our professional narrative includes the vast experiences, skills, and knowledge of all nurses, what will the future of nursing look like? As a historian and informaticist, we cannot predict what is to come, but the Nurses You Should Know project makes clear that the future of nursing is in our hands.

References

Creative Reaction Lab. (2022). *A method for co-creating equitable outcomes*. https://crxlab.org/our-approach

Hao, Y., Liu, H., Yue, S., & Liu, X. (2011). Introducing traditional Chinese nursing: A review of concepts, theories, and practices. *International Nursing Review, 58*(3), 319–327. https://doi.org/10.1111/j.1466-7657.2011.00918.x

Hunt, D. D. (2017). *Fast facts about the nursing profession: Historical perspectives in a nutshell.* Springer Publishing Company.

Lengstorf, J. (2018, May 21). *Make the right thing the easy thing: Designing processes teams will actually follow* [Video]. YouTube. https://www.youtube.com/watch?v=xqT8e6_yzLg

Lewenson, S., & Herrmann, E. Krohn. (2008). *Capturing nursing history: A guide to historical methods in research*. Springer Publishing Company.

Nurses You Should Know. (2022). *Medium*. https://medium.com/nurses-you-should-know

Seltzer, J. (2021). Andrés Fernández. Nurses you should know. *Medium*. https://medium.com/nurses-you-should-know/andrés-fernández-420a749cbddd

Smiley, R. A., Ruttinger, C., Oliveira, C. M., Hudson, L. R., Allgeyer, R., Reneau, K. A., Silvestre, J. H., & Alexander, M. (2021). The 2020 national nursing workforce survey. *Journal of Nursing Regulation, 12*(1), S1–S96. https://doi.org/10.1016/s2155-8256(21)00027-2

The Voice of Advocacy: If Not You, Then Who?

Adrianna Nava, PhD, MPA, MSN, RN
2021–2024 President, National Association of Hispanic Nurses

I have seen women of color crack, break, and shatter glass ceilings at the national level. Most recently, my heart was overfilled with joy to see Judge Ketanji Brown Jackson make history as the first Black woman confirmed to the US Supreme Court on April 8, 2022. Despite this historic achievement, I could not help but also be bothered by the persistent reproof of her professional record during the confirmation hearings. "These bad faith efforts exist despite a resume that arguably surpasses those of previous nominees," stated the Chair of the Congressional Black Caucus (Sprunt, 2022). The fact that women of color who are qualified, or many times *overqualified*, must continually prove that they belong in positions of leadership can deter Black and Latina women from entering the leadership pipelines at local, state, and national levels. National level leadership is essential to advocating for health equity, addressing structural racism, influencing national policy agendas, and inspiring future generations to be agents of change. But how do we get there?

In my 12 years of nursing, I have sought out opportunities to lead within the Veterans Health Administration and the National Association of Hispanic Nurses (NAHN). In these roles, many times I was the only Latina in a room full of leaders. I knew this needed to change, and I was compelled to spark interest and propel more Latino nurses into policy and leadership-oriented fields. This will not only increase the diversity of the nursing profession, as we strive to look more like the people and communities we serve, but also prepare more Hispanic nurses to seek national leadership positions.

Policy, leadership, and advocacy go hand in hand. Effective policymaking is needed to keep organizations, staff, and patients safe. However, without leadership and advocacy, policies often do not consider disparities due to race/ethnicity or socioeconomic status and mainly focus on overall system performance. Although headlines in health disparities related to COVID-19 made waves, until we fix the incentives within our healthcare system to focus on rewarding not only overall quality but also quality for all sub-groups (whether it is by race or socioeconomic status), then we are not really invested in improving healthcare quality and out-comes for everyone.

> "A nurse's voice does not need to be the loudest or most dominant in a room. We must be more concerned with the way our voice resonates—with intelligence, integrity, grace, and passion. As advocates for health equity, a nurse's voice speaks for more than the individual, it speaks for those who depend on our message to enact change, and that is a power we must be emboldened to use."
>
> –Suzanne Miyamoto, PhD, RN, FAAN
> Chief Executive Officer, American Academy of Nursing

America, which is composed of "[a] nation of organizers" (Gross, 2016, p. 4), is well suited for nurse leaders to build collective action to improve the health of our nation. One way is to participate in a national nursing organization and become involved and visible. It is uncommon to see nurses being called to national leader-ship positions or presidential appointments, but I know we belong there—along-side physicians, scientists, and politicians. By participating in a national nursing organization, you are placing yourself at the intersection of leadership, advocacy, and policy—the perfect place to gain experience in leading change and the perfect place to take a stand on the disparities that many in our country suffer from. We know that nurses participating can make a real difference in advancing health equity.

Since 2011, I have held various leadership roles within NAHN to build my technical and adaptive leadership skills as a millennial nurse, since it was difficult to navigate into a leadership role within the traditional work settings. As the 2011–2013 President of the Illinois Chapter, I led the growth of the chapter from a network of 20 to one with over 200—the fifth largest NAHN chapter in the country by the end of my term. From 2014–2016, I was elected to the NAHN National Board of Directors. In this role, I oversaw membership growth and initiated, proposed, and saw passed the amendment of the NAHN bylaws to create a category for unlicensed healthcare personnel to be welcomed into the organization as affiliate members. This category of membership is vital to NAHN's mission, as many Hispanics work as nursing assistants or medical assistants and should be encouraged, through adequate mentorship and access to resources, to continue their education into nursing.

In Boston, I became the 2015–2016 Vice-President of the Massachusetts Chapter. There, I created the Nursing Leadership Scholars Program to focus on providing Hispanic students and nurses training on community leadership development. In this 10-month pilot program, I mentored six nursing mentees who learned about their role as nurses in health policy. Through the program they (1) received education on leadership and health policy over the summer, (2) organized a Hispanic health fair in June 2015, and (3) developed two professional development workshops for nurses in our local community. Individually, the participants reported improved communication skills and increased self-confidence via the program evaluation. In addition, two healthcare fellowships and four nursing school scholarships were awarded, and two participants were elected to the executive board of the NAHN Boston Chapter (with one of them being elected president).

In July 2020, I was elected President-Elect of NAHN, my first national leadership position. This is when I realized the significant impact I had on the lives of others. My mission up to this point has been focused on elevating the profession of nursing and the Latino community so that we can be active participants in healthcare policy decision-making. Both groups are dramatically underrepresented in positions of leadership and influence in the United States, leading to policies that result in poor health outcomes for Latinos and poor working environments for nurses.

Although advocacy at times is voluntary, this experience has shaped who I have become and has opened many doors of opportunity for my members and me. On April 4th, 2022, I was deeply proud to be invited by President Biden to the signing of the Executive Order for Strengthening the Affordable Care Act and Medicaid (see Figure 10.1), with the honor of representing hundreds of Hispanic nurses. I share my leadership story with you in the hopes that you will continue your journey and reach out to organizations that are here to support and propel you forward.

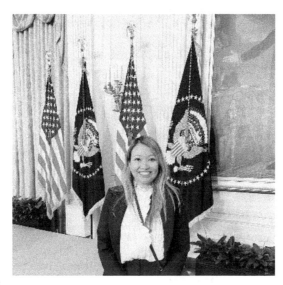

Figure 10.1 NAHN President, Dr. Adrianna Nava, at the signing of President Biden's Executive Order for Strengthening the Affordable Care Act and Medicaid.

References

Goss, K. A. (2016). *The paradox of gender equality: How American women's groups gained and lost their public voice.* The University of Michigan Press.

Sprunt, B. (2022). Judge Ketanji Brown Jackson confirmation hearings: What happened Thursday. *National Public Radio.* https://www.npr.org/2022/03/24/1088492365/judge-ketanji-brown-jackson-nomination-hearings-what-happened-thursday

Won't Give Up

Music & Lyrics Written by Tad Worku

Tad Worku is a songwriter, singer, speaker, and nurse practitioner. His music is available via most music streaming services. You can find out more at tadworku.com.

V1
Sometimes the road is lonely
Sometimes it's hard to do
And if you feel you're the only
Listen up I wrote this song for you

You know your road's been trodden
And someone's walked in your shoes
And when you feel like it's over
Oh no it's just the start of chapter two

CHORUS
So keep on knocking
Love keep on walking
Even when it's hard to do
And don't you know dear
You'll make it home here
Cause love it won't give up on you

V2
Sometimes the world is heavy
Sometimes it breaks you down
And when your knees ain't steady
You'll find your strength when they hit the ground

CHORUS
So keep on knocking
Love keep on walking
Even when its hard to do
And don't you know dear
You'll make it home here
Cause love it won't give up
No it won't give up
Said love it won't give up on you

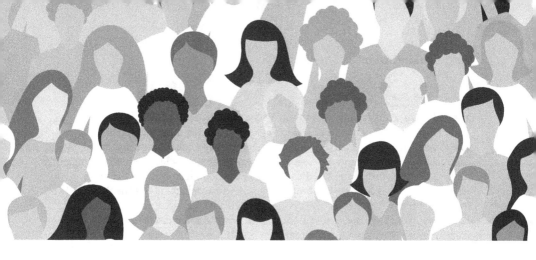

History as a Guide to Envision a More Equitable and Just Future

When I was asked to contribute to the Afterword for *Taking Action: Top 10 Priorities to Promote Health Equity and Well-Being in Nursing*, the most recent edition of *The Power of Ten*, with a specific focus on the history of health equity and structural racism in nursing and how the nursing profession has addressed these things in the past, I was torn. After all, the nursing profession's history of addressing structural racism is admittedly complex, and there are debates about the degree to which nursing has been actively involved in efforts to address structural racism. Some have called out the seeming passivity of nursing when discussing structural racism. Others have pointed to examples where the nursing profession has been at the forefront of advocacy, activism, health promotion, and efforts to address health inequities.

To be fair, there are legitimate points on both sides of this argument. The American nursing profession is plagued by a legacy of racism. At the same time, the ugliness that racism represents in both society and nursing stands in contrast to many superlatives attributed to nurses such as "caring," "nurturing," "healers," "trusted," "advocates," and "activists." However, if structural racism is defined by the way our systems' resources and services are structured to advantage and disadvantage one group over the other, then the history of the nursing profession provides an exemplar case study of its presence at every level of practice, education, regulation, and research.

Indeed, just as structural (and interpersonal) racism impacts the lives of millions of historically marginalized people, through segregated living conditions, limited access to high-quality healthcare, and opportunities for employment and education, its pernicious effects are also evident in professional nursing. By taking the time to identify, interrogate, and reflect on the ways that nursing has been complicit in perpetuating disparities, while highlighting those who resisted and prevailed against these injustices, we stand to uncover viable solutions rooted in our past.

No, history is not a blueprint for addressing structural racism, but it can be a teacher, illuminating our individual and collective power to dismantle, redesign, and rebuild health and professional systems that are rooted in justice and equity.

The Past as Prologue

As a discipline, professional nursing emerged within the late 19th century and in most ways reflected the deeply rooted racial animus echoed in many quarters of society at the time. Black nurses were barred from admission to nurse training schools in the US South, and in the North, quotas were introduced to reduce the number of racial and ethnic minoritized trainees (Hine, 1989). Professional nursing organizations, including the American Nursing Association, required nurses to join via state nurses' associations, effectively excluding minoritized nurses given that most state nurses' associations denied them membership (Bennett et al., 2019). Advanced training opportunities were also limited for minoritized nurses. The education of nurses in midwifery, for example, reveals the ways in which public health nurses and physicians joined forces to eliminate Black and immigrant midwives, while refusing nurses of color admission to nurse-midwifery training schools (Dawley & Walsh, 2016). In light of these seeds sown in our past, it should be no surprise that we are reaping the harvest of racial health inequities, especially Black maternal morbidity and mortality.

Some would like to believe that the plague of racism that marks nursing's legacy is in our rearview mirror. On January 25, 2022, the National Commission to Address Racism in Nursing (2021) released the results from a survey of over 5,600 nurses with findings showing nearly 65% of Black nurses reported experiences of racism, while another 63% of nurses reported that they have personally experienced an act of racism in the workplace. That survey was conducted not in 1961 but in 2021, suggesting that structural and interpersonal racism in nursing is not a function of our past but is reflective of our present-day reality.

The choice of response is ours. Will we acknowledge our past and confront our present-day reality with passive indifference or with a steely resolve for change?

Centering the Margins & Applying Lessons Learned

In my own quest to find evidence of change agents who were addressing structural health inequities, I was introduced to a nurse pioneer, Mary Elizabeth Tyler. During my days as a doctoral student studying health disparities in early 20th century Philadelphia, I learned that Tyler served as a central figure in a successful health campaign to fight tuberculosis in low-income Black neighborhoods in Philadelphia beginning in 1914 (Brooks Carthon, 2011). To her credit, Tyler linked her care not to the presumed biologic inferiority of Black Americans but instead toward social conditions such as poverty and a lack of health information. She would go on to make hundreds of home visits and serve as host to numerous community health lectures (Brooks Carthon, 2017). In the end, she helped facilitate a significant increase in community engagement with local healthcare centers by leveraging community affiliations and addressing social needs. If reducing health inequities begins with addressing the social determinants of health, then we should do more to highlight Mary Elizabeth Tyler and others like her. Tyler's largely unknown biography offers a master class on leveraging a community-informed, strengths-based approach.

Like Tyler, Henrietta Villaescusa (1920–2005) worked throughout her life to improve the health of Hispanic/Latino community members. She obtained her nursing degree, public health certificate, and master's degree in the mid-1940s. After holding various nursing positions, Villaescusa went to work for the Los Angeles City Health Department, earning a position as its only Hispanic supervising public health nurse. She served as a member of the Centers for Disease Control's Hispanic/Latino subcommittee for the National Diabetic Education Program. As Chief of Citizen's Affairs, Office for Economic Opportunity, she established innovative nationwide community participation programs for the Office of Health Affairs. She was the first Hispanic person to serve as the bureau's Federal Women's Program Manager and the highest-ranking woman of Mexican-American parentage in the bureau (*Pasadena Star-News*, 2005). If health inequities are differences in health between and within groups of people caused by socially structured, marginalizing conditions, such as unjust laws and policies, then Villaescusa's leadership at the federal, state, and local levels demonstrates a multi-level approach for advocacy and activism.

Finally, throughout her lifetime, Dr. Mary Elizabeth Carnegie (1916–2008) worked to increase educational opportunities for nurses from diverse backgrounds. In 1943, she established the Hampton University School of Nursing. She also served as the Dean of the School of Nursing at Florida A&M and successfully fought to desegregate the Florida Nurses Association. To her credit, Carnegie carefully documented the contributions of African American nurses in numerous books and articles including the widely acclaimed *The Path We Tread: Blacks in Nursing Worldwide, 1854–1994* (Carnegie, 1999). In doing so, she sought to amplify the voices of those who were most marginalized. If our goal to address health inequities includes diversifying the nursing workforce, then Carnegie's life's work demonstrates the strategies and tactics needed to fight systems of exclusion, while centering nurses from diverse backgrounds whose contributions to the profession and health activism are often left at the margins.

Envisioning Our Transformative Future

Reflecting on the lives of Tyler, Villaescusa, and Carnegie reveals that we each have a role to play in combating structural racism and ensuring health equity, whether in our communities, work settings, professional organizations, or politically. Our fight, like theirs, begins by acknowledging that we cannot dismantle structural racism without acknowledging that structural inequities are an artifact of our professional and social history and are embodied in our practice, policies, and personal and societal attitudes. At that same time, we must honor our predecessors by anchoring our legacies to the strategies that forged their activism and picking up the mantle to push nursing to harden its commitment to equity.

In her groundbreaking poem, "The Hill We Climb," poet laureate Amanda Gorman encourages us to fight injustice through collective bravery, even when the weight of structural racism feels like too great a burden to bear: "When day comes we ask ourselves, where can we find light in this never-ending shade?/The loss we carry, a sea we must wade./We've braved the belly of the beast./We've learned that quiet isn't always peace, and the norms and notions of what just is isn't always justice./And yet the dawn is ours before we knew it" (Gorman, 2021, pp. 11–13).

Indeed, the dawn (future) of nursing is ours. If hopelessness is the tool of the oppressors, then we must fight the urge to give into apathy or exhaustion because the stakes are simply too high. We must imagine the nursing profession in radically inclusive ways—ways that force us to deal with the discomfort that arises when we discuss racism because we are unpracticed; radically inclusive ways that encourage accountability because as problem solvers we must do more than talk the talk, we must be committed to walk the walk even when the path we tread is difficult: "For there is always light, if only we're brave enough to see it./If only we're brave enough to be it" (Gorman, 2021, p. 29).

–J. Margo Brooks Carthon, PhD, APRN, FAAN
Tyson Family Endowed Term Chair for Gerontological Research
Associate Professor of Nursing | Secondary Appointment, Africana Studies
Associate Director, Center for Health Outcomes & Policy Research
Chair, Graduate Group in Nursing
Executive Director, THRIVE
University of Pennsylvania School of Nursing
Department of Family & Community Health

References

Bennett, C., Hamilton, E., & Rochani, H. (2019). Exploring race in nursing: Teaching nursing students about racial inequality using the historical lens. *OJIN: The Online Journal of Issues in Nursing*, *24*(2). https://doi.org/10.3912/ojin.vol24no02ppt20

Brooks Carthon, M. (2011). Making ends meet: A historical account of community networks and health promotion among Blacks in the city of brotherly love. *American Journal of Public Health*, *101*(8), 1392–1401. https://doi.org/10.2105/AJPH.2011.300125

Brooks Carthon, M. (2017). Minority nurses in diverse communities: Mary Elizabeth Tyler and the Whittier Centre in early 20th century Philadelphia. In S. Lewenson, K. Smith, & A. McAllister (Eds.), *Nursing history for contemporary role development* (pp. 3–18). Springer Publishing.

Carnegie, M. E. (1999). *The path we tread: Blacks in nursing worldwide, 1854–1994*. Jones & Bartlett Learning.

Dawley, K., & Walsh, L. V. (2016). Creating a more diverse midwifery workforce in the United States: A historical reflection. *Journal of Midwifery & Women's Health*, *61*(5), 578–585. https://doi.org/10.1111/jmwh.12489

Gorman, A. (2021). *The hill we climb: An inaugural poem for the country*. Penguin.

Hine, D. C. (1989). *Black women in white: Racial conflict and cooperation in the nursing profession, 1890–1950 (Blacks in the diaspora)*. Indiana University Press.

National Commission to Address Racism in Nursing. (2021). *Racism's impact in nursing*. https://www.nursingworld.org/~48f9c5/globalassets/practiceandpolicy/workforce/commission-to-address-racism/infographic--national-nursing-survey_understanding-racism-in-nursing.pdf

Pasadena Star-News. (2005). *Henrietta Villaescusa obituary*. https://www.legacy.com/us/obituaries/pasadenastarnews/name/henrietta-villaescusa-obituary?id=26841230

CPSIA information can be obtained
at www.ICGtesting.com
Printed in the USA
BVHW050825190223
658800BV00015B/1174